Fitness Is A Mind Game

Fitness Is A Mind Game

How to Lose Weight &
Get Your LIFE Into Shape

A Book About Life Fitness Management

Dr. Glenn Mollette

Acknowledgements

Thanks to every person who has ever made a contribution to my spiritual, mental and physical well being. The list would be almost infinite. For ministers and teachers and basketball coaches and exercise friends who have always encouraged me to go for the best. Without your mentorship and guidance the right path might have been a little more difficult to find. But God has His way and His way meant bringing you into my life. Thank you.

Before you begin any kind of exercise/physical fitness program –
talk to your doctor!

Chapter 1

Starting is the Hardest

Any program to slim down and shape up is hard to start. It's hard because it is such a lifestyle change. Even if you have dieted and exercised many times before, you are asking your body to go through it again. You have stepped on the scales and said to yourself, "Oh no I weigh far too much." Or, the dreadful morning comes when you arise to discover those trousers are no longer tight – they will not even fasten. Your thought is, "I have to do something." But the question is what are you going to do? What are you really going to do?

The answer for many is to head off to the mall to buy new and bigger trousers. Soon, those trousers are filled to capacity and the dilemma becomes …what next? Buy more and bigger trousers? Or do you make that radical decision – start trying to shed some weight. Sometimes it's like a war inside your mind. You truthfully want to be leaner. You want to feel healthier. You hate the miserable bloated feeling that keeps you from seeing the person in the mirror that you want to see. But this person you want to see in the mirror is so far away from existing. How far? 50 pounds? Is it more like 100? Or, could it be only 30 or 40 pounds separates you from the person that you can only imagine seeing in the mirror?

What are you going to do? The answer is getting your body and life in shape! And you say, "Sure…I'm going to start…tomorrow." Tomorrow comes and you feel tired, stressed or have too much work to do or too many errands to run and you put what is important on the back burner. You are important, and day after day if you are not extremely careful you will put yourself on the back burner. Neglect is one of the harshest treatments of all.

When you don't take care of yourself the price that you and your family pay is incredulously high. Don't think you are doing anybody any favors if you allow your health to diminish by not taking care of your weight problem. You are only allowing a scenario to develop that will take the life out of your family a little later down the road. People who do not take care of themselves are creating a liability for their loved ones. Individuals who carry too much weight and treat their bodies unmercifully will reap unkind rewards. We reap what we sow. The reaping will be in the form of diabetes, high blood pressure and other life threatening problems that will require doctor's visits and tons of medication.

The most physically fit people in the world get sick and die. Fitness is not a voucher for eternal life. Fitness is an admission ticket to feeling good until you do die. The chances are on your side that if you are fit you might extend your life a few years and feel good while living!

Some people live to be 80 and feel bad and limp along every year of their existence. Some people live to be 80 and they are invigorated, enthusiastic, pleasant, lean and productive. Make a choice. But don't wait until you are 80 and then say, "I want to be the lean, productive person." I'm not saying it's too late to start at an older age. We all want to believe it's never quite too late. But why not enjoy your life and add some real life to your years? You can.

Reading a book such as this required a start. You picked it up and began to read. Getting your life into shape is all the same. You begin. You begin today. You say okay, "I'm going to do it." You say, "I can do it." You don't know for sure how long it will take you but you know that you can do it. You know that you can drop the pounds and get your life into the kind of shape that you have been dreaming of for a long time

I want to help you. I want you to use what God gave to you

– your mind. Yes…your mind! In this book we will discover the unlimited source that you have within you to make your life and body what you've been able to only dream about. The mind has the incredible ability to make choices. The mind may choose dessert for the hand to reach out to and put into the body. Or, the mind may say, "The dessert looks so good and so pleasing to my eyes. But I know how it will wear on my hips or stomach and so I'd better take the salad or vegetables instead." The mind may prefer the sugary taste of three or four soft drinks a day but is able to discern if I cut out that sugar intake and drink water, or beverages without the sugar, then I have a chance of fitting into my dress or suit.

The mind is that part of you that makes the call on starting this new life and new you. This is the hardest of all. The hardest part of walking or running a mile is making the decision to put on your shoes and go out the door. Once you have started then you are on your way!

Starting requires us to say, "Today I'm going to eat properly. Today I am going to eat less fat and less sugar. I'm going to cut my calorie intake to the number that it takes for me to shed a pound or maybe even two a week." In the meantime you are confronted with gut wrenching obstacles, food on every side and every excuse imaginable to not exercise.

Let's do it. Let's start. Let's start together. I am with you! There is always a need in my life to lose five pounds or make an adjustment. Almost every day I need to anew and afresh my commitment. Yesterday's decisions have to be reaffirmed today. Just because you said twenty years ago that you would always love your wife or husband doesn't mean that you don't renew your love and commitment daily. Life is daily.

You probably have started a thousand times. Let's start again. Let's start by saying, "I'm going to do it. I can do it. With the strength God gives to me and the mental fortitude that He has placed within me I can start to move forward with becoming fit and shaping up my life!" You made this same statement and vow yesterday? Good for you! Make this same commitment today. Even if you failed yesterday, you likely did not fail as much as you might have had you not made a vow to work on your life.

Every day you start because every morning is a new start! Even if you were very successful yesterday and the day before, don't count on yesterday's success carrying you through today.

We fail on many days because we are living in the victory of yesterday and allow today to blind side us. We ate the amount of intended calories and walked the two miles and feel so good about how successful we were that when the breadbasket is passed we rationalize and say, "I can have two rolls because I was so good yesterday." The result of this kind of let down is a messed up day that we end up regretting because we let our guard down.

Daily we start.
Each morning we get out of bed.
Each day we set ourselves in motion.
If there is no beginning there is no completion.

While you may not have started yesterday, you must start today. Because if you do not start today then another day of this wonderful life that God has given to you is wasted. Maybe, it is not totally wasted…but all that your day could have been, did not reach it's full potential. All it required was a start, because once we start our chance of finishing is better. People who run races are much more apt to finish the race than those who never even approach the starting line. While there are those who begin races and never finish, their accomplishment is better than those who never tried.

An old adage is true, "It is better to have tried and failed than never to have tried at all." But the wonderful aspect of this life that

God has given to us is that we get to try again and again and usually many times.

I have lost weight and gained it back and then lost it again. I do not have a body that is naturally thin or highly metabolic. I envy some of my friends who can eat all they want and never gain a pound. That's not me. I can eat all I want and the next day it shows on the scales and my waistline. I can be careful about what I eat and exercise and lose the weight or I can be unscrupulous and put the weight on. Every day I must choose. I must choose between what is good and bad but also between what is good and best.

There are many good choices. Why not choose the best?

The choice between good and best is likely choosing one helping of food over two helpings. It is choosing to walk a couple of miles verses two hours on the couch watching television. While two helpings of food or resting on the couch watching television is not necessarily bad they are not the best for you in comparison to healthier options.

Since life fitness requires us to start each day anew and afresh and can be a battle, let's do the following:

1. Start and start right now. I understand the big dessert is in the refrigerator or a big dinner for you to sit down to is in the works. But you can't put off life impacting decisions. You put it off and then it is put off again to where you just totally forget about it. Have one spoon of the dessert if you have to and say, "Mmm that's good! But I'm tired of feeling bad and fat, so, this dessert must go into the trash." Or give it to someone who can better afford to eat it.

    You may go to the big dinner, but before you sit down at the table, make a decision about how much you are going to eat. Take small portions and take few portions. Keep it to a couple of items. No, you cannot eat a little of everything. If you take a little of everything on the table you will end up with one big plate of food! Big plates of food result in big meals that result in weight gains. Start and start right now to work toward life fitness!

2. Ask for help. Many times I've had to say, "God I need your help." We are not gods who have unlimited abilities. We are human beings who are very capable magnificent creations. We have amazing abilities. Yet, we are frail. We have battles. We have struggles. We wrestle with decisions. We sometimes make bad choices that hurt us. We need help from on high. Daily we are in warfare making decisions about what is good or best for us. We are pulled to the right and to the left. Ask God to help you. Many times I have said, "God I am failing. I am eating like a pig. I have no control when it comes to buffets. I have not exercised in two days. Please help me today to do what is right."

3. Make a mental decision. Your decision is within you. It's between God and you. Support and exercise friends are very helpful…but the commitment comes within you. Only you know how you want to feel and look. You can't ask somebody, "Do I look okay?" What are they going to tell you? They are going to be diplomatic and say, "You look fine." They are not going to be honest and say, "Gee, you look awful. You need to lose 50 pounds." People for the most part don't want to hurt your feelings, so they lie to you telling you what they think you want to hear. You must decide within you what you want to do. You mentally say,

"I want to lose the 30 pounds. I detest how it makes me feel and look! It's not about anybody else but me. I'm doing this for me!" Reach within you and make a mental decision!

4. Evaluate the reward. The reward determines our level of enthusiasm and commitment. A paycheck increases the determination to get out of bed and go to work. You may love your job but if there was no salary you couldn't do it. You go for the financial reward. The reward of fitness is you. You are the reward. At the work place you strive for your employer. You are financially benefited, which in turn enables you to pay your rent. When you start working toward life fitness, you are working for you and the results are multiple: appearance, how you feel, confidence and ability to be more productive as an employee, spouse, parent or whatever you enjoy doing.

5. Incorporate life planning. A Life Fitness Planning Pad will help you put down on paper what you weekly and daily want to accomplish in your life.

START NOW!

Chapter 2

Life Fitness

There is nothing better than when everything is working!
Take for example your car. We love a car where everything is in
order. We drive down the highway and the motor moves us along
at whatever speed we are allowed to drive. The transmission is
working. The brakes stop us for the traffic and red lights. The
headlights and taillights are working as well as the instrument panel,
radio, windows and seat adjustments. The tires are properly balanced
allowing us to enjoy a smooth ride.

But take one of those away. For example the headlights go out.
Darkness comes and it's impossible for you to navigate your way. You
can't find your way. Other cars will not see you and you will likely
be hit. You become a danger to others on the highway. Suddenly the
car has a problem that desperately needs to be fixed – the headlights!
Even on rainy days your car is disadvantaged because you need the
light to enable others to see you.

You look at your car and you love it. You like the paint job.
You like the style. You like the ride when you are cruising at 65mph.
The stereo system is quality. You are proud of it. There is just one
problem – your car is now limited. It is limited to daytime driving
only because the headlights don't work. With the many hours of
darkness in a 24-hour cycle your car will idly sit waiting for the sun
to rise.

Of course, the way to solve all of this is to fix the headlights.
You take your car to your dealership and repairman and you have
new lights installed. The sun sets and you are once again on your
way to driving at night. It was so very simple. A simple procedure

made the scope of your driving life greater and much more enjoyable.

Our lives have some similarities to a car that is only partly in working order. Our bodies age and become frail and reach a state where it's difficult to keep everything operating smoothly. The body ages and dies and returns to the dust of the earth. Cars become scrap metal to hopefully be recycled in some fashion for further use. Yet while both are in operation overall maintenance is a must.

Life is more than one entity. Jesus said, "Love the Lord your God with all your heart and with all your soul and with all your mind and with all your strength." (Mark 12:30). Jesus recognized that life is more than just sheer physical strength. He recognized the importance of our inward selves. God wants a body that glorifies Him but God is dishonored when we say we are giving our bodies to Him but our hearts and minds are not into it.

A husband and wife give their bodies to each other. But in marriage the mutual exchange of each other's bodies is hollow without love. What makes the marriage union so marvelous is not two physical human beings living in the same house but the mutual sharing of heart, soul and mind.

Sadly, some marriages today are united only in strength. The day-by-day life is more physical endurance, requiring sheer strength to survive or even cope with the marriage union. This is not a very fit way to live. The marriage needs mental and heart help. Without it, the marriage is not going to make it.

A 1000 piece puzzle is a beautiful picture when all the pieces are properly joined. But when there is a piece missing in three of four sections, then the whole picture is not complete.

Life fitness is letting all the pieces fall into place. This does not rule out adversity. This does not exempt us from pain or pressure. This does not mean every day is a mountain top experience. Beautifully running cars drive through valleys and over mountains. They face rain and drive in the snow. They look great in the sunlight but move ahead when the roads are slick and hazardous. Because they are in proper running order they are able to operate in the harsh conditions as well as the good.

As persons we operate better when life is fit. A fit life is a better-suited life for peace and joy. For example, let's say you have great job skills and an education to match them. But you are so overweight that you truthfully are not performing your job like you could if you were not so loaded down by this extra weight. Maybe you are doing well in spite of your condition. How could you perform if your heart didn't have to work so hard to supply blood to your body? A leaner body will give you an extra boost of energy. Don't you deserve that? At 3:00 in the afternoon when you have already put in a full day yet there is still so much to do – don't you need and deserve a little extra spark as you face the house, the kids, supper, homework and so much more?

A life that can point to many diplomas and certificates and educational attainments surely feels a sense of accomplishment and satisfaction. But it's not enough. I have seen too many medical professionals walking the hallways carrying an extra hundred pounds or even much more. I don't want to hurt your feelings, but if you are a doctor or nurse you must get your body into shape. I've heard of doctors being 50 pounds overweight and talking to patients about the need of losing weight. The patient receives mixed signals. The patient thinks, "Wait, you are an obese medical professional and you are telling me to lose weight?"

I've seen far too many nurses and nurse's aids that physically were not able to help the patient because they couldn't bend over to assist the sick patient on the bed. Therefore they preferred to sit behind the nurse's station desk and tell other aids what needed to be done.

I've seen too many doctors and nurses and other medical professionals standing in the smoking areas of the hospital sucking every inch of a cigarette into their lungs before walking back into the corridors of the hospital to render – medical care? Imagine how much greater impact these medical persons could have if they took greater care of themselves physically.

There are many people who are physically limited by disease or debilitated by accidents. It could be you are one of these people. My wife was limited to a wheelchair for over eight years before she died from the ravages of multiple sclerosis. While her body became unable to do anything she was still able to touch people's lives with her spirit and wisdom. She couldn't do what a person having the use of all of his/her faculties can do, but she greatly contributed to life, family and friends. For her, it seemed like one headlight was missing along with two of the wheels. Yet she worked with what she had and strove each day to do all she could to make each day the best that it could possibly be.

That is all that we can do. Trying to do our best is all God ever expects. God does not expect us to do what we cannot do. He only expects us to do what we can do. It's when we don't even try to do what we are humanly able to do that we get into trouble.

We can try to take better care of ourselves. We can try to lose the extra weight that is short changing us and depleting us of energy. We can make an effort to overcome the bad habit that is dragging us down.

On the other hand, exercising and dieting all day can become a real rut. I have friends who spend three or four hours in the gym five days a week. That is a lot of your life and time. If you are training for an athletic contest then it could be necessary. But if you have other responsibilities such as vocation and family or other interests then you can't spend that much time in the gym or exercising. You don't have to.

If you spend all your time working out every day then how productive are you at work? Are you too tired to do your job because you have so drained yourself? When you come home from your workout do you not have anything left to give to your wife/husband because you spent yourself on the treadmill or in front of the mirror lifting weights?

Too many people make decisions to lose the weight, then they go for a couple of weeks or even months pushing themselves as hard as they can but burn out and think, "What's the use? I'm dead tired all the time and have not lost much if any weight." Or, they are shaping up but their whole other world is crashing around them.

What good is it for you to get your body in shape if everything else fails around you? Don't throw your career and loved ones away while you pursue the perfect body. Instead, keep it all intact. You can have a good career, healthy relationships with loved ones and a body that is in shape.

That's what you want isn't it? Of course you do. We don't allow ourselves to verbalize it but in the heart of every person the desire to have it all exists. We just get frustrated in life and quit imagining it to be possible. We settle for the least and quit dreaming and working for the most. We become accustomed to looking at our fat selves in the mirror. We don't allow our minds to wonder back to a time where we wanted to be more active and productive – maybe even leaner and healthier feeling.

We do this in so many other areas of our lives. Education and training is so very important. We have a bad semester or do poorly in a class and think, "It's just too hard." The mind grows tired of pushing and trying because failure is exhausting. Many people settle for less education because they quit imagining that they can finish the course. Sometimes it's special training. Or, it may require four or even eight years of grueling study. Why would you ever think that you couldn't do it? Maybe you can't today. But maybe you can start envisioning a month or a year when you can begin the journey on whatever road you want to walk. You may be at an age that seems inappropriate. Please…get over age. Age is only a number. There are some eighty- year- old people going to college and other kinds of schools. The mind is ready when you are.

Life fitness is a package deal. Life fitness is your effort to complete the puzzle. Life fitness is like the finely tuned automobile running smoothly down the interstate.

Nobody is perfect. No life is perfect. No body is perfect.

The human body always requires maintenance…proper nutrition, exercise and many times in life medical care.

The human mind is a marvelous organ that God has given to us. The mind can be used for good or bad. If we allow our minds to be dominated with negative, ugly thoughts then it will send these negative, ugly thoughts throughout our bodies. The body can only respond as led by the mind. Your body cannot do good deeds if your mind is not thinking good deeds. Your body has the ability to be ugly and be an evil to society if led to be such by your mind.

Jesus realized how important it is for us to have victory in our internal lives. A glorious body begins with a glorious mind. He said, "Love God with your heart, soul, mind and strength (Mark 12:30).

There is no strength to love God if the mind and heart are not into it. Our minds send the message to the body that says, "This is good. This is right. This is something that will feel right or proper. Therefore go for it!"

Fitness is a lifestyle.
Fitness originates in the mind and extends to the body.
Fitness means planning daily for a great day.
Sow a thought reap an act.
Sow an act reap a habit.
Sow a habit reap a lifestyle.
Sow a lifestyle reap a destiny.

Take control of your body and your life by taking control of your mind. Determine that your mind is going to be healthy and productive. Utilize your heart, soul and mind to be channeled in the proper direction.

Chapter 3

Go To Bed

There is no strength for exercise nor the ability to think clearly if you are exhausted. People today go through the motions of life sleep deprived. Before you even try to think about moving ahead with trying to get your life into shape, you should go to bed and get some sleep. You probably need a lot of it.

Too many people today brag about going to bed late and rising early. They brag about how much they had to do late into the evening while arising early to tackle the day. They think they are getting ahead of the game by working so hard. Sadly, this mentality puts you far behind.

People are lethargic while needing ten cups of coffee to seemingly see them through the day. We live in a world where people are edgy, easily agitated, and coarse in their conversation to family and fellow workers. Road rage is epidemic. People get huffy over the smallest matters. Could it be we need some sleep?

You want Life fitness? You want to look better? Get some sleep and get sleep every 24-hour cycle. Truthfully I can't sleep eight hours out of 24. If I sleep seven I have done well. However, I firmly believe in power naps. The power nap may last from five to thirty minutes. I don't think I've ever slept more than 20 minutes in the afternoon. But, it is amazing how much better I feel the rest of the day even if the nap only lasted five minutes. This all depends on what is going on in your life mentally and physically. If I am sleeping seven hours in a night and am physically lean I seldom need a nap.

Most places of employment would gain far more from their employees if they allowed them a 20 minute space of time to completely feel free to sit down, drop their heads and go to sleep. When they awakened they would have more energy to face their tasks, plus a clearer mind.

How many people do you see each day with their faces about to fall off from lack of sleep? Maybe you are one of them. When you are sleep deprived you eat more. You are more prone to be in the refrigerator hunting for a snack. You think you are hungry. Actually what you are doing is trying to compensate for your lack of rest. You think food will make you feel better and while a few more carbohydrates may give you a little boost you are still sluggish. If you are tired almost every day and eating a little extra to compensate for your weary feelings, you are only creating another problem – excess pounds. The excess pounds multiply. Now you are not only tired from lack of sleep, but also tired from carrying excess pounds. The excess pounds cry out for more food. The bigger we become the more we want to eat. It develops into a negative lifestyle.

When you are sleep deprived you cannot sufficiently exercise. Exercise makes me feel better and perky. Yet, I do not exercise properly when I am in need of sleep. I may go through the motions of running a couple of miles. I may limp through a routine of weight lifting. I may halfway do an aerobics class, but I am not maximizing my time efficiently.

Our total beings hinge on how well rested we are to perform the task. A wise man once said, "I have so much to do I must go back to bed." You have to face a group of people and make a presentation? You need to be rested so that you can be alert to clearly present your material.

You have to put in an eight or ten-hour grueling shift of work? Go to bed early. You will not be productive if you are exhausted. My father was a coal miner and for many years worked nights. We had a small building behind our house where he slept most of the days. There was no way he could survive working in an underground coal mine without mentally being sharp and rested to face the challenges of coal mining from the 1940s through his retirement in 1975. He had no choice but to get sleep.

As a child, I can remember an irritable daddy if, during the summer time, I awakened him with the sound of a bouncing basketball. Most people are irritable if awakened from sleep especially if they know they need to be rested for the next day.

Fitness is a mind game. You are going to lose the game if you are too tired to play it. You are not going to do well at work, at home, at the dinner table or in your exercise program if you have not had enough sleep.

You will also come up short in your thought life. Your thought life permeates your body. The thought life sends happy messages or negative messages to the body. Your thoughts say, "Legs you can run three miles." Or your thoughts may say, "I'm so tired I can barely get through the house."

If it is your day to walk or run three miles and you didn't sleep enough last night, then try to squeeze in a 20-minute nap. You will awaken a little groggy but in another twenty minutes the cobwebs will begin to clear and you will have more interest in pursuing your run.

A very self righteous person once was challenging a group of Christians about how they were not working hard enough in their Christian service. He tried to become eloquent and said, "The devil never rests." One wise man said, "Yes that is very true. And if we never rest then we will become just like the devil."

A strategic part of life fitness is rest. Plan to be good to your body and rest adequately.

Chapter 4

The Battle for Your Mind

Never have there been so many books, fitness machines and fitness television programs. We are submerged as never before with sleek looking men and women on television showing us how we can look if we will only fork out the cash and buy a certain machine. This machine, just barely used a few minutes a day, will have us looking like the model in just a short matter of time – we are led to believe.

Pills are promoted today as being the answer to fitness. Pills are pushed and we are promised they will cut our appetites and the pounds will just drop off.

We are shown exercise routines by dynamic personalities. These routines will give us the body of our dreams if we will only purchase their videotape and follow the patterns on the tape religiously. I think there are many great exercise tapes and instructors on tape but are you going to watch this tape five days a week? I seldom enjoy watching a movie more then once or twice. What do we do after we bore watching the same tape a dozen times?

All kinds of foods are marketed today as the answer to health, fitness and weight loss. If we only drink or eat a couple of these small portions a day and eat very little at night we are promised weight loss, better appearance and fitness. These products work – for a while. However, they are not your lifelong answer. Let's get real...do we really want to spend our entire lives relegated to a canned drink in the morning and one at lunch and almost nothing to eat at dinner? We do not, we don't and we won't. We try for a couple of weeks and sometimes much longer, but it gets old. Soon the mind begins to view this daily routine as very unappealing and you quit because we grow to despise eating this way.

Have you ever thought about how limited we have allowed ourselves to become in attaining life fitness? We have allowed our options to be relegated to a few machines sold over the television. Or, we have plugged into a couple of diet plans, promoted by huge industries, that make the foods they want you to buy from them. Or, we have adopted an exercise program or two we watch on television but that soon fades, as we cannot always be in front of the television.

I think this is why so many people reach a point where they almost try not to think about losing weight and life fitness. So many don't know what to do next. They may have bought one exercise device after another and tried one diet after another only to find themselves right where they where three months before.

Fitness is a mind game. Fitness is not going to happen because you shelled out $39 and now you have a device in your closet or under your bed. It's not going to happen because you have spent $200 on pills that were advertised to melt your fat away. Fitness is not going to happen because you changed over to diet beverages. Actually some diet beverages make me hungry. You must change your mind. Change your mind. Change your body. A fit body is a result of a fit mind and planning weekly and daily to make life fitness your daily agenda.

What does the average television infomercial do for you mentally? The average infomercial treats you and all of us like we're stupid. We are told all we have to do to look great is try their product. We are shown a picture of some guy who has lost 100 pounds walking toward a fast food restaurant with a big smile on his face and the message is - if we do what he did we will lose the same amount of weight too. Really? Who wants to eat at the same location twice a day for a year? Even if following this regimen works, what do you do after you have lost the 100 pounds? You can very easily put it right back on. If you are not careful, you may gain back more than a hundred pounds, and that is surely the last thing you want to do.

We have so many mixed messages in the media that battle for our minds. One commercial may promote a diet drink while the next commercial is promoting super sized fries and greasy hamburgers made with three slices of cheese. We have become so confused that we are apt to sit down with a can of Slim Fast to drink with our Whopper.

My grandmother was a sweet wonderful Christian lady but surely was a hundred pounds overweight. Diet wafers were a fad during her day and I remember her eating a few of these along with the big dinner that she had fixed for grandpa.

So very much else today contends for our minds and what occupies our minds may determine our eating and exercise habits. Mentally, we eventually reach a zone where some of the messages we receive do not even faze us. We soon learn that we cannot drink sugar filled soft drinks and eat cheeseburgers every day. Pizza smells and looks good, but Pizza is not the right course for weight reduction. The milkshakes our kids enjoy can only be a visual enjoyment for us most of the time.

I certainly believe that if we periodically want a milkshake or a slice of pizza, we are entitled to it. But, we can't make eating like this a lifestyle.

Restaurants are creative at marketing their desserts. Some of them look beautiful and we can imagine how tasty they would be too. But we have to take note how that dessert will look on our backside or our waistline because that's where it is going to end up.

We eat more today than ever before. Restaurants give larger portions than ever. Most of the people I associate with eat more than I do. Unfortunately for me, I have some friends who have high metabolisms and can eat twice what I eat without it affecting them. There have been times when I have been to lunch or dinner with them and they are eating like horses and mentally it's very easy to think, "I'll just join in." But I know my body and how much I can eat. Since I know what I can and cannot do then it is only reasonable that I do what I know I can do. It's when I do what I know I can't do that I get into trouble.

We violate ourselves when we go ahead and ignore our sanity. If we know that 2500 calories of food in a day is going to add a little weight then why would we eat 2500 calories three days in a row? We might get by with it one day a week or even two if we are exercising a lot and burning the calories.

My body will lose just a little weight every day if I maintain a 1700-calorie intake. I can maintain my weight at about 2000 – 2200 calories a day. If I begin to go above that and I am not running or exercising then the weight gain is going to occur. I know …it sounds miserable to have to be this meticulous about how much I can and can't eat. But it is what I know. When I know something, then I can either deal with it or ignore it. To ignore it would only be crazy for me.

There is something within us that cries out for us to ignore the truth. I don't know what or who it is. Maybe it's just our human nature to try to ignore truth and reality. We do this all the time. We try to put off planning our funerals. We say, "I'll deal with this at another time." We try to put off making out a Will. Again we say, "I'll deal with this at another time." Yet both are very important for us to personally handle, before life changes and we cannot have a part in handling them.

People want to procrastinate making spiritual decisions. A spiritual decision to become more dedicated in our walk with God or more committed to any lifestyle that requires some attention and discipline, is something we know to be worthy of thought. We say, "We will get around to it."

Maybe it is the devil. The Bible speaks of the evil one who was always at work in the Bible to bring about chaos and destruction. This same evil one is very alive and well in our world today. I think he often appears in subtle ways and his ways of destruction are not always bold. A human life can be rendered incapacitated with more than drugs, immorality and other bad habits. A human life can become enslaved to food. Instead of being in the gutter of life saturated with booze we can be perpetually in the easy chair with a sack of donuts or a bag of candy. While we may be able to legally navigate our cars after consuming a half a dozen Twinkies we are still painfully out of control

Eating is the Christian's sin. For too long, Christian people have laughed about this and then gone right on ignoring it. I have known far too many big fat preachers. Some of them have been very precious dear friends to me. They lived very good lives and were very committed to God and were faithful in their calling. Yet, while their sermons were good their appearance preached a louder message. Their appearance said, "I'm out of control in my life." How can a person be a man of God and be so out of control in his life?

The Bible speaks of the fruit of the spirit being self-control. Check out Galatians 5:22. While we may hide some of our sins we cannot hide the sin of eating like a pig. It shows all over us.

Some Christians mask their anger. They put on a good face in public but then storm all over the house in front of their family. A Christian may piously hide his/her selfishness and other sins that are not easily spotted. But a Christian cannot hide his gut.

We can't be perfect. I'm not saying that it's humanly possible for us all to have flat abdominal muscles. Men and women both battle these areas respectively. But what we are to do is to mentally be aware of our lives and who we are and what we are doing with and to ourselves. Instead of being stupid and ignoring the truth, mentally, we become conscious of ourselves and we respond accordingly. We can still very much enjoy life. It just means that if you have a 600-calorie breakfast and a 700-calorie lunch that you had better be very careful when it comes to the last meal of the day. You must make a mental note to be careful because you are about to get into trouble if you eat an 800-calorie dinner.

This is not grueling painful work that I am talking about. I am talking about having power over your life. Instead of allowing media messages, mental pictures and other subliminal messages to control us – we control us. We control who we are.

We control who we are.

We control who we are.

We control who we are. Say it this way. "I control who I am."

We are faced with much in life that changes our course and alters much of what we do. Adversity and valleys come our way if we live long enough. But with every problem we can still be who we want to be. Life is not being who you are. Life is about being who you want to be. Who you are is not a constant given. Who you are is what you choose to become. It is what you plan to become. Weekly and daily planning moments result in achieving life's goals.

We sometimes say, "I am who I am." No you aren't. You are who you planned to become. You truthfully may be the son or daughter of John Doe Smith. John Doe Smith may have owned a bakery and produced the finest cakes in your town. You will always be the physical child of John Doe Smith. But you don't have to grow up to run the bakery…unless you want to. Nor do you have to enjoy cakes the way your father enjoyed making or even eating them.

I have enjoyed writing most of my life. I wrote my first A+ paper while in the seventh grade. It was humorous poem about "The Night Before Christmas," that was an assignment for junior high class. While I was in high school I used to write little papers and envision them being books. When I was 23 I made my first failed effort at writing a book.

When I was 24 I was hired to be a journalist for a state Baptist paper that had a circulation of about 50,000 and kept that post for ten years. In 1998 I made a decision to write "Silent Struggler: A Caregiver's Personal Story," which is the story of caring for my invalid wife. My writings have been mentally decided choices. While people have been nice and encouraged me to write, I had to make the choice. Within my mind I had to make that mental commitment. Writing comes easy for me. Yet, it is because I want to write. I think anything we want to do comes easier.

I am a writer because of choice. I plan weekly and daily to write. I am not who I am. I am what I choose and plan to become. I was not born a writer. Nobody in my family that I know about writes articles or books. You are not a doctor, salesman, factory worker or mother of six because that's who you automatically were but because it's what you chose to become.

We all make mental choices that we regret or are happy about, but choose we do. It's tragic when we begin to believe that we cannot choose. If we begin to think we cannot choose to exercise, eat right or lose weight then we have mind work to do. Don't forget what this book is about – Fitness is a mind game. Most of the battle for a fit life is the exercise program that is going on in the top section of your body – your mind. For you to be convinced, in your mind, that you have to carry an extra 100 pounds or more and that you can't change your life, is a mental devastation.

Why would you think this? Are there family members who have convinced you that you are stuck with all this weight? Do you have a circle of friends who have made you believe that you have to stay fat in order to be their friend? Has the idea of trying to get your life into shape made you believe that it's unspiritual or wrong? What has you in mental gridlock? Are you afraid to try? Are you afraid

of failure? What makes you stuck in your circumstances? Someone
or something or some past experience has likely trapped you into
mentally giving up and just being fat and unhealthy.

Mentally, it can be a battle. There is a battle for your mind. But
guess what? It's your mind. God gave your brain to you. He even
let's you make your own choices – good or bad. God wants want is
the very best for you but He did not make you a robot. You have to
choose between evil, good and even what is best for you. Friends
may tell you what is best and fat preachers may convey conflicting
messages and mental images that you see and hear over the
television. But who do you want to be? Take control of your brain.
Choose this day who and what you will be.

Chapter 5

Mind and Body

A healthy body is a blessing. You can make it in life if you have God and a healthy body. If you have health you are very rich. If you have a relationship with God plus good health you have it all.

What do you need for completeness in this life? You need the void in your inner life met and that void is like a hole that only the love and grace of God can fill. Next, you need health to adequately do this life. If you lose your health, God is there for you in the good days and bad. He has a place beyond this life prepared for every believer in His Son. But doing much in this life requires a body that will enable us to perform the tasks of life.

Lose your health and you are limited in what you can do. You may compensate in other ways, but dwindling health can only be compensated so long. A person who becomes wheelchair bound may still participate in races...but races of a different kind. A person who loses an arm may still function in life with one arm but there are difficulties that come with having only one arm. A person who loses a foot can no longer do what the person with two feet can do. The scenarios are endless.

So much of what happens sneaks up on us. A car wreck is almost always an accident that could leave our bodies permanently altered. A birth defect is not something that anyone asks for but does his/her best to deal with the hand of cards that has been dealt.

There are people who inherit physical problems. My niece was diagnosed with diabetes in her very young adult years and underwent a kidney transplant by her late thirties. There is a history of diabetes on her father's side of the family. A good friend started battling heart problems in his mid thirties. His father died of a heart attack when he was fifty and his grandfather died of heart failure at a younger age. It seems that when there is a family history of heart problems, they are passed from one generation to the other.

Yet, we live in a world where billions have been born with bodies that had all the necessary essentials to have long, healthy productive lives but abused their bodies to the very death. The body is strong and works hard to survive. The body is amazing like nothing else that God ever made. Yet even the best body can only take so much abuse.

People who continue to smoke while taking chemotherapy for cancer is amazing to me. What are they thinking? Guess what…they aren't thinking. They aren't thinking about their health at all or they would quit smoking.

I talk to people fighting diabetes. They take insulin injections every day or a pill. The doctor has warned them that they could lose a foot or a leg and they eat everything they are not supposed to eat. They do not exercise and they are slowly abusing their bodies that will end in death of the body.

Granted…the body eventually dies. But you don't have to push your body into the grave fifteen years ahead of schedule. Plus, why destroy the quality of the remaining years of your life?
You might use the last fifteen years of your life for travel, adventure, rewarding charity work or just enjoying your grandchildren. God made this world and saw that it was good. It is good, if you have the health to enjoy it.

You can have multi millions of dollars but what good will that do if you don't have any health. Sure, you can pay the doctor's bills if you have lots of money. But if you have your health you can work until you are 90 years old and even older if you want to.

I have talked to many senior adults in their seventies who could make it without working twenty hours a week but they find it mentally good for them to have something meaningful to do. Their work enables them to get out of the house, talk to other people and to keep their bodies in motion.

Our local paper once did a story about an 86-year-old man who delivered pizza. Maybe he had to have the money for his livelihood. But, he was able to do the job. I met the man and I was impressed that he was moving in and out of his car as well as I do.

An 88-year-old man in my community drives every day and farms. He seems to enjoy life. He is bodily able to do life and has a wonderful attitude and disposition.

For purposeful living we must make a concerted effort to care for the body. Slothful, abusive living only rewards us with disability. We reap what we sow. If we abuse the body the toll of our blows will soon be evidenced in our diminishing health.

Cancer, heart trouble and other health problems can arise even when we have done well to care for ourselves. But they will arise sooner if we flagrantly put on ourselves what is not good for the body.

So why do we do to ourselves what is bad? Why do we go without rest? Why do people smoke cigarettes constantly? Why do people intoxicate themselves with alcohol time and again? Why do people have random sex? Why do people work twelve hours a day? Why do people eat every meal like it is the very last…packing their bodies with food until it is coming out of their ears? Why do people not exercise at least a little? It's a mind game.

Mentally we allow ourselves to not think. God has given us brains that we do not maximize. It is interesting that some of the smartest people on the planet can be great scientists, surgeons, educators and public leaders and treat their bodies like garbage. It is especially interesting today with all the knowledge that has been made available to us about health and how to have healthy lives that people ignore proven information.

Mentally we succumb to the smallest matters. We have power

at the office for eight to ten hours but cannot stop putting food in our mouths. We have power on the assembly line but cannot control a negative pattern of behavior that we fall for after work.

You are in control. You may not be in control at this very moment. But you can choose to take control of your life. Life fitness is you stepping forward and determining your daily life and choosing your destiny. God has given you the power to choose. If you choose a life of victory and health He will help you.

"I can do all things through Christ who strengthens me" (Philippians 4:13).

There are habits and negative lifestyles that become addictive. Over eating becomes a negative pattern of destruction. The other habits and addictions that tear us down are endless. There are times when we find ourselves lost and needing help to pull ourselves out of the swamp of despair and destruction. God is our helper. He never made us to walk off and leave us without help. We can choose to go our own way. We can choose to try to do life without God. But why would we? God made for us this incredible place. He made us and knows all about us. He knows what makes the body work to its greatest ability. He knows how to make us completely happy and at peace. Why would we want to ignore this awesome creator? When we allow the distractions of life to throw us off our course God is there to help us back on track and to keep us going in the right direction.

Mentally we choose. We choose life. We choose to pursue health as long as it is available to us. We choose to make the selections that will enhance our health and enable us to have long quality lives. These right choices can only have a positive impact on the body.

The body does what the mind tells it to. Take charge and lead your body in the right healthy direction.

All along the way we have God. God is our helper.
Struggling a little to get on track? Feel overwhelmed?

Do you feel like you are too far gone to make a turn around in your life? I have one word to say to you, Never!

This doesn't mean you can make the NBA basketball league if you are 50. Nor does it mean that you can bring back a dead child from the grave – at least in this life. But it does mean you should never think you are too far - gone to take hold of your life.

"If God is for us who can be against us?"(Romans 8:31)
God is for you.
Right now say it, "God is my helper. God is for me. I can do it."

Chapter 6

Imbalance is a Miserable Life

One of the stumbling blocks to life fitness is imbalance.
An imbalanced tire prohibits us from cruising comfortably on
the highway. We can drive on the road with all the tires being
imbalanced but the sheer fun of driving is made almost impossible.

Life can be almost impossible at times. Often the reason for this
is because of the imbalance in our lives. We live in a time where
people feel they must be going five directions at once or they are not
doing anything.

A parable was told once of two angels that where watching
planet earth from a distance. They looked at all the movement
and activity and one said to the other, "Where are all those people
going? The other one said, they aren't going anywhere, they're just
going."

We can easily become a life that is going, but going nowhere.
I have been around people who felt it was important to be busy
regardless if any mission or purpose was being accomplished. It's
important to have something to do. But whatever we do should add
a certain dimension of quality to our lives. When we do too much it
is likely going to create imbalance.

Too Much Exercise/Too Little Exercise

It can happen. While this book is about life fitness, fitness is
more than four hours of exercise a day. Spending two hours on a
treadmill is unnecessary. Yet, I have seen too many people feel that
their only hope to happiness was full mornings of constant exercise.

They are doing it wrong. Their life is out of balance. Granted, someone may be striving for the Olympic gold medal or preparing to run the Boston marathon. Such contests and sports events call for extraordinary training. But even the greatest of athletes will burn out if all they are doing is exercising. Sports figures and professional athletes obviously incorporate their fitness programs into their livelihoods. They represent a tiny fraction of the world's population. Much of the world is juggling jobs, family, church, hobbies and exercise. Few of the world's population have the time to exercise three hours every morning. People have other things to do like the laundry or the kid's baseball games.

Exercise can happen. Good exercise on a daily basis can happen. But it doesn't have to happen at the expense of you not functioning in the other areas of your life.

On the other side of the coin is too little exercise. We very easily are consumed with jobs and family and school and hardly have time to give exercise a whimsical thought. When this happens we are hurting ourselves. We are subjecting ourselves to a severe penalty. The failure to exercise is creating body inability. We are allowing an imbalance to occur in our lives that eventually will incapacitate us and keep us from enjoying life to the fullest.

It is up to you to determine how much time you can spend in an exercise program. Only you know how much time you have and how your body is responding.

You can figure a minimum of twenty to thirty very active minutes five to six times a week for a successful exercise program. Once you are conditioned you can run two miles in twenty minutes. Or for twenty to thirty minutes you can do a very brisk walk.

Too Much Food/Too Little Food

We will say this several times in this book. Eating all the time creates horrible problems. Our bodies don't require that we feed them constantly. While you may eat several meals every day they cannot be but very small meals. If you eat three big meals a day you are going to carry a lot of excess weight. If you eat one very big meal a day you are likely going to carry a lot of excess weight.

So much of eating today is "want" and "desire." Our eating today is not based so much on what is good for us or what our body needs. We want the cookies, the snacks, the chips, the cheesecake, the two or three soft drinks, the greasy cheeseburger, the loaded pizza, the salad with extra cheese and lots of dressing. This kind of eating adds up to fat, fat, FAT! It becomes an imbalanced ride to destruction.

I'm not saying you can't eat a cookie or a piece of pizza or have a slice of cheesecake. But it had better be done in moderation. You had better balance it out in your life. A slice of cheesecake a day will have you literally rolling around the house like one big ball. You don't need dessert every day. Save it for once or twice a week. Make Friday or Saturday night your celebration night. You have worked very hard during the week and you have either maintained your weight or even lost a pound or two. You can allow yourself to have a sliver or small dessert. Don't go hog wild and eat the biggest dessert in the restaurant or that you can create. Be rational.

Too little eating is just as bad. If you cut your food intake back so far then you don't have the fuel you need to do life. You have to eat and eat regularly. I like the idea of grazing several times during the day. I eat a very small breakfast at about five or six in the morning. By ten or eleven I am ready again for a small meal. By noon I like to eat again and then another snack at three, five or six and then eight. Six very small meals a day is a reasonable plan. You plan for these eating times. You know that at planned moments you are going to eat! You plan exactly what you are going to eat. This cuts down on all of this out-of-control late night eating. Sometimes

I'll have a scoop of vanilla ice cream at the evening meal. But, it all depends on what I've had during the day and how much exercise or activity I've had.

If you cut back your eating to almost nothing then your body's metabolism slows down to compensate for your eating pattern. Instead of burning fat your body begins to store whatever fat it can save because it feels it is going to need it to survive. Don't be so bad to your body. Give your body what it needs to function. Fire needs fuel. Your body will not burn fat without the fuel. You can develop a balanced daily pattern of eating that will give your body what it needs and will even allow you to lose a little weight every week. You will see results and feel like exercising and being active. Once you get into balanced eating you will feel so much like exercising and being active that it's going to amaze you how much you have been missing in life.

Too Much Play/Not Enough Play

The imbalanced life affects every aspect of living. When was the last time you gave yourself a day to do something fun? You could be burning yourself out by your too much work lifestyle. You may be someone who works nine hours a day and then goes home to another shift of cooking, cleaning, kids and a schedule more rigorous than your paying job. Somehow you must find a way to play – at least some. A fit life will consist of a schedule that permits a day for some kind of hobby or recreation. If you don't have it you are going to explode. It may be a hobby, exercise or craft project. But everyone needs some type of release.

Yet I know people who spend too much time playing. Their whole lives consist of extracurricular activities and therefore they are robbing themselves of productive living. They are not doing well at their jobs and nothing is getting done at home but all their evenings or spare time is spent in playtime.

I suppose the analogies of imbalance are endless. One that may or may not apply to you is Too Much Church/Not Enough Church. There is such a thing as going to church too much. If you feel that your religion requires you to be out of your house and at your place of worship or religious service four or five times a week then you probably are focusing on religion and not a relationship.

Too often people become religious about having to be at church every night of the week. A part of life fitness is attending a place of worship. Our spirit has an inner craving to be fed. The Bible tells us "Not to give up meeting together, as some are in the habit of doing, but let us encourage one another" (Hebrews 10:25). But it doesn't mean that we are to attend the functions of the church to the point that we do not have the time to be husbands to our wives or wives to our husbands or parents to our children. Some churches offer services in addition to the Sunday morning service. This is a call each person has to individually make. There may be weeks you need worship two or three times. There may be weeks that Sunday morning or Wednesday night or Saturday night is all you can attend.

This analogy pertains to your service to all civic organizations or extra-curricular activities.

Guess what? God gave you a brain – use it. You know how much you have on your plate and what you and your family can do. I've seen people gripe about having to be at a series of church services for three or four evenings. They would say, "We don't have the time to be here. Or, something else is going on that I should be attending to. Then, attend to whatever it is.

Don't go to the buffet and gripe all evening about how much food you are eating. Don't go to the buffet.

Use the mind God gave you.

There are times when you would like to be someplace but you can't. There are times when you would like to eat more but you know you shouldn't. There are times when you would like to be at the special Thursday evening gathering of some organization but it's not feasible for you.

Balance is not always possible. Too often we try to cruise down the road totally out of balance. We are going forward but the ride is rough.

Try balancing your life.

Chapter 7

Have Fun It's Life

Why does fitness and trying to physically shape up burden so many people? People everywhere speak of diets and new plans they are trying with almost a sense of dread. I hear stuff like, "I'm starving." Or, "I hate this diet I'm on." Or, "I don't have enough energy to get out of bed in the morning because of this low carbohydrate diet I'm eating."

People look at fitness programs as if it has to be some morbid, serious daily ordeal. If your doctor has told you that you are going to die very soon if you don't lose a hundred pounds then it definitely throws a serious twist to your exercise demeanor. But attitude is everything and so you need to have fun with whatever you need to accomplish. When exercise and life fitness is enjoyable it's much easier to pursue.

There are days when you are running, or working out hard that you may not be smiling but you will when the workout is finished and you see the results of your efforts. Stepping on the scale seven days after serious proper eating and serious committed exercise will reward you with numbers that will delight your life.

1. Consider how seriously boring it is to be miserable. When you cannot bend over to tie your shoelaces. When you have to huff and puff to get out of your chair. When you cannot put your favorite trousers or dress on because you are too fat then you feel bad. Who wants to live this way? Is this any way to live if you can change it?

Not all of life can be changed. People live with birth

defects and handicaps from accidents; and sickness renders some people to limitations that can never be reversed. These people who take hold of life and do the best they can with whatever they have left are courageous heroes.

How sad it is when so many people have minds and bodies capable of changing their course in life yet sit idly watching four hours of television a day. I talk with people who spend a lot of time being depressed. They want to have hours and hours of counseling. They want somebody to constantly talk to them and try to make them feel better. What most of these people need to do is get into motion and pursue life.

Everybody can stand instruction and advice on how to handle adversities and problems. Everybody needs someone to talk to. But there comes a point where the individual must mentally decide he or she will do something.

Why not decide that you are not going to be miserable? You say, "You don't know my situation." God does. "And we know that in all things God works for the good of those who love him, who have been called according to his purpose" (Romans 8:28).

My wife was a total invalid for several years. She could neither walk, nor feed herself. She could do nothing for herself. While I would have done anything possible to change her situation I did not die to depression and care giving. I thank God for her multiple sclerosis. Yes…sounds weird and almost totally crazy to say those words. But mentally it's better than saying, "I hate God for her multiple sclerosis."

Hate is a very draining, debilitating emotion. Hate and anger render us sick and useless. A person filled with daily anger and hate will end up very physically sick. An attitude of thanksgiving is a lighter load to carry. It's a happier load. I mentally and consciously choose the lighter load.

Don't get me wrong. Caring for someone with multiple sclerosis or any kind of debilitating disease is tough. Mentally it can drain you, sling you in ten directions and toss you aside on the scrap heap of life. It can…if you let it.

With every scenario of life we must find a way to win. Battles are lost but the war is what we want to win. Daily we may lose a battle here and a battle there but the overall victory is the ultimate goal.

When we are in misery the battle is already lost before we arise to the challenge. We are zapped of the energy to take hold of the tasks at hand. Being miserable is boring.

2. Dark rooms were made for light bulbs. I've never seen a dark room that couldn't benefit from a light bulb. I can't imagine building a house without lighting. After all, in the wintertime it becomes dark so early. I can't imagine sitting in the dark or trying to eat in the dark in the evening time. Nor can I imagine any homeowner taking all the light bulbs out of his/her house. People do it to their lives.

Sadly people almost willfully turn all light out in their lives and live in darkness. Regardless of your intuition and sense of direction it's hard to move forward in the dark. You can't drive in the dark. You can't read in the dark. You can't see what you are eating in the dark. Darkness is a bleak place to do life successfully.

Before we can have life fitness, we have to do something that may be at first painful and that is, turn on the light. Turning on the light reveals more than we may want to see. But we can't deal with what is allowed to hide in the dark.

Often, turning on the light and looking at our selves in the mirror can be scary. It reveals a body that needs some work. But often when we turn the light on in our souls it can reveal attitudes and emotions that are subtly making a very negative impact on our lives.

Take a good look at your inward life. Do you have feelings or emotions of anger, hate, jealousy, insecurity or lack of trusting someone that are robbing you of your happiness? What good are they doing you? How is having any one of these feelings making you a happier person? How are they making you better? They aren't. They are making you miserably boring.

3. Life was made to live. When you are bogged down with internal misery you don't feel like living. You don't feel like walking the three miles. You feel more like sitting on the couch with your potato chips and watching time-consuming television programs. God gave us life to live. You can't live well when the life is filled with internal darkness, bogged down with baggage that is making your life very difficult.

Internal Junk

Freedom to enjoy life and to pursue happiness comes about
when we turn the light on in our lives and exam ourselves
internally. Finding out what is going on inside, enables us to
address it, deal with it and overcome it. Fitness is a mind game.
Mentally, we allow ourselves to lose the battle of internal
junk. Internal junk zaps us from making it to the gym or robs
us of eating healthy. We pout, live in depression, and become
dysfunctional to the normal routines of life. Again, misery is a
very boring way to live.

Mental Image

What is it that you would like to have? You want a happier life?
You want a better marriage? You want to be a better parent? You
want to do better in school? You want a better, healthier body?
Draw a picture of what you want. If you imagine it you have a
chance of achieving it. Success begins with an idea.

"Where there is no vision the people perish" (Proverbs 29:18).

We never accomplish our goal because we lock out a proper
mental image of what it is that we really want. We are fearful
of visualizing a fit body. We dare not imagine eating right daily.
We can't imagine our lives being fit and feeling good about who
we are. We allow ourselves to slip into mediocrity. We sigh,
"I'm doing as well or better than some people." We compare
ourselves. While it is nice to admire people we should never
compare ourselves because we are all different. I cannot do
what many do, but I can do what I can do. What I can do is

what I should do. What I cannot do is a waste of my energy to think about. Yet, what we can do is more than what we allow ourselves to imagine.

We suppress our imaginations, dreams and desires. A vision of being better than what we are can sometimes be troubling. We briefly allow ourselves to see the vision but then quickly turn it off. Why? Because the vision will require hard work, patience, time and likely making sacrifices that we don't want to give.

A couple wants to buy a house. In order to buy the home they will need a down payment. The down payment will require sacrifice. Certain pleasure items may have to be put aside in order to accumulate the financial goal. All the time the mental picture of owning the house is in front of them. The sacrifice is worth it because they know within time they will have their house. The house is the mental picture of what they are striving for.

Mental images are goals and goals are good for us all. A goal gives us something to aim for. Every arrow needs a target. The marksman becomes skilled with his rifle because he practices shooting at a target.

What is your target? What are you aiming toward? What is your vision? What is your goal?

Without a goal you will perish.
Without a target you will hit nothing.

Life was made for us to live. Internal junk and life without vision only make life more difficult for us to enjoy.

4. Who told you life couldn't be fun? We allow the circumstances of life to steal our fun and happiness. It's not always easy to be happy every moment of the day. Our happiness is based so much on events or happenings. Happenings are always changing and therefore it is reflected in our demeanor and countenance.

    But if you don't learn to have some fun in life, some day you are going to be one old crusty bitter person. Fun doesn't require that you do anything immoral, illicit, illegal or unbiblical. Just be like Jesus. He was the most awesome guy in his day and time. He was the life of the party. He turned water into wine and saved weddings, broke up funerals by bringing dead people back to life. He fed the hungry masses when nobody else could. Jesus – what a man!

    The best friends I have to this day are the people that I had fun with. Doesn't that make sense to you? Your dearest friends are those people you trusted enough to let your hair down with. People that you have to guard against saying the wrong thing will never be close to you.

    Sadly, this is why most people in most churches and places of worship never get to know their ministers or staff. Nor, even more sadly …one another. On average they feel too insecure to be relaxed and say and do as they might in an informal situation. There is great pretense. Pretense isn't fun and is very unhealthy.

We do this at most places of employment and many vocational settings. We only act as we feel we are expected to act and perform. Question...isn't that miserable?

A happy life is a real life.

To this day the people that I was just completely real with are the people that I continue to correspond with and remain friends. Life has to have some fun. You cannot be fit in body and mind if you have convinced yourself that you cannot enjoy life.

I maintain a balanced exercise program. But there are times when I even deviate from my schedule. Just this past Saturday my two sons and I spent the day on a pontoon boat. What were we doing? Goofing off. Jumping in the water and driving it as fast as we could up and down the lake; which probably was never more than 20 mph.

Sometimes our church brings loud alternative Christian bands into the gymnasium area of church. Our kids jump up and down to the music and there are occasions I jump up and down and carry on with them. My two kids recently wanted to see one such band in St. Louis. We made the drive and I stood in the balcony with all the other old people. It was loud and it was fun. About three nights after that we attended a Billy Graham crusade in Louisville, Kentucky. Billy Graham had an incredible line up of alternative type music. I have never seen so many teens and adults getting into the music and having so much fun.

Life fitness will not happen if you do not learn to loosen up. If you stay tense and uptight you are going to harden and break apart.

Chapter 8

Beware of Negative People
And ...the Negative One
(Mind Drainer)

Life has enough difficulties without having to overcome negative people – sadly they are a reality of life. No matter how positive life is there always seems to be a negative person lurking somewhere close by.

The negative person can always find a reason why it can't be done. He sees the barrier to every success and the reason why something good is going to go bad. He can't imagine how any mountain of adversity might ever be removed. He will always find a reason why you can't or why you shouldn't. He can put a slant on anything that you are trying to do in your life that will make you think twice about doing it. Sometimes the slant is a little chuckle that says, "Oh what you are doing is silly." Sometimes it's a little shaking of the head and rolling of the eyes that is a subtle method of putting you down for your effort. Often it's the questioning, "Why are you doing that? What makes you think you can accomplish that task? Who do you think you are to make such an effort?" Beware of such people.

If you know that a person is truly negative to the core then you can handle them a little better, which is by avoiding them as much as possible. Often these people are our closest associates and avoiding them is totally impossible. Since we can't avoid them then we need to have some built in mechanism of protection.

When you arise in the morning with a strategy of how you may better do life, how you might make the most of your day and are then confronted with negative associates, you need a plan. You can begin every day beaten and defeated if you keep company with people who constantly see the flaws in your life and not the sunshine.

Most of us see our own flaws and know well of our imperfections. We don't need a lot of professional daily commentary to make us feel worse than what we already do.

There is a plus to having a good friend that cares enough about us to tell us the truth. It is true there are people who only tell us what they think we want to hear. A good friend who loves us enough to say, "You are really messing up in this one area of your life," can be a real jewel.

If this good friend says this to us about every thing in our lives we are doing then likely you need to find another friend. Not everything you are doing is wrong. It takes a wise person who can spot the good and the bad and discerningly offers input that will make a positive important difference in your life.

Fitness is a mind game. Every day, the mind makes decisions about eating the right food and carrying out the proper exercise program. Some days it's a battle of the will. A company of negative people around you will make your battle even worse.

1. Beware of the overweight person who tells you that you don't need to lose weight. Really? How are they making this determination? Are they basing this comment on what you really want for your life and what you feel you need or are they comparing you with them? Chances are they have not made a mind and heart commitment to pursue life fitness and it is driving them crazy that you are trying to become mentally involved in your life. Be nice to these people but don't ask for their input. Better yet, don't tell them what you are doing because it only opens a door for them to start

talking to you. Often it will begin with a silly question, "Why are you doing that?" Or, "Why do you want to do this?" They have not personally come to the place where they have made a decision and your decision means you are ahead of them in this area of life.

2.   Beware of questioners. This is the friend or associate who wants to know why you are taking an exercise class or why you have gone to walking five miles four times a week. Asking a question is one thing, but it's another when the question is toned in such a way that it comes across as more of a statement than a question. The question may come across more like, "You are silly for doing that." But the silliness is with them for asking such a question.

Negative people can drain you mentally. When you think you are ready to proceed with a plan, they have a way of spotting a weakness in the plan. There are few perfect plans for life fitness. Gaining control of our lives is the best plan that is available. Daily and weekly planning out our eating, exercise and life achievement goals is a monumental forward step. We have a marvelous God who helps us and is available for us. God gives us the power to make choices and we control our destiny. He will empower us to do what is right or we can go our own way.

The Bible tells us the devil lurks in the world and he is the author of destruction. He brings about destruction to every situation where he is allowed an opportunity to work. He is not only the evil one...but he is the negative one. In the very beginning of time he was giving Eve unsolicited advice about what was really best for her. What he convinced her of wasn't good for her or anybody else. He is still doing the same today.

He works to deceive us. When he does, we are impacted along with all others that our lives encounter. He led her to believe he knew better than God. He is still at work today giving people unsolicited advice.

Daily he will feed you with negative thoughts. The list is endless:

- "Stay in bed and don't go to the gym."
  "Don't go jogging."
- "You don't need to lift those weights."
- "Aw forget those abdominal exercises. You can do those later."
- "Hire the grass mowing people to do your lawn. You are too busy to get out there and push that lawn mower."
- "Go to the donut shop and eat some donuts."
- "Go have a couple of sausage biscuits with cheese instead of doing your thirty minutes of exercise."
- "Just let yourself go. You can start an exercise program after Christmas. But between now and Christmas just eat whatever you want." (And of course gain the fifteen pounds that it will take you ten months to shed...or never shed).
- "You have a career and a job right now. You had better put all your mental energy into what is going on at work. You can always think about exercise at a later date." (Of course what happens is that you begin to feel so bad physically that you can't perform well at work).
- "Yea, of course you should exercise...but you need to be cooking meals for the kids. After all, you are their mother and they need to eat." This is so very true. You want to feed and care for your kids who are always hungry. But you can't eat everything they eat. This is when life gets real tough. It's a battle to have good food

in front of you when you are trying to limit your
intake. Of course, this is the very key…you have to limit
your intake of what is available. Plus, if you don't get
your exercise you are not mentally going to be the able
mother that you want to be. Your thirty minutes of hard
pumping exercise clears some of the mental cobwebs and
sweats some of the poisons out of your body.

Let's face it negative people and the evil one are realities. They
both exist. Mentally they can drain us of the internal energy that we
need to be effective in areas that are personally beneficial to us.

Life fitness is a personal endeavor. It is about you. It is about
you being the best you can be mentally and physically. When you
are the best you can be, mentally and physically, then you are in the
position to be the best daddy or mommy that you can be. You are
more able to be the kind of spouse that your husband or wife needs.
When you are take care of yourself you are able to better care for
others. If you have neglected your mind and body to the point that
you are falling apart, what do you have to offer those you love and
care about?

The destructive ways of this world are so wise. The evil one
and the forces of negativity play colossal tricks on us. The device
used is that we don't have time to take care of ourselves because
of all the other commitments we have. We use our energy to fulfill
every other commitment and ignore ourselves. When we ignore
ourselves long enough then it begins to take its toll. We become
sluggish physically. We gain weight. We become less able to fulfill all
those commitments that we had prioritized above ourselves. Soon
most of them become such dreaded chores that we have to give
them up or fail at them. We soon begin to lose our health because
we have ignored our health. As health diminishes, then life and our
mental health diminish with it. Then, the devil has us right where
he wants us – out of commission and unable to contribute all that

we could have contributed had we not been deceived by his lies and negativism.

Every human being has a great deal to offer the world. Every life can make a difference. So many people work very hard at doing their best. The only hope the devil has is to diminish us. He wants to diminish our lives to where we are less effective or not effective at all. An ineffective life becomes a dismal life for the person who once was so effective.

Sow these thoughts today. I want to be the best person I can be for my spouse. I want to be the best I can be for my family. I want to be the best I can be for my vocation or career. Therefore, I must be the best that I can be for myself. If I am not the best I can be for myself then how can I ever be the very best for the people I love and the career I want to do effectively?

Fitness is a mind game. Don't let the evil one and negative influencers in the world deceptively drain you of what is important. Plan daily for effectiveness!

Chapter 9

Mental Exhaustion

Life fitness encompasses mental care. Mentally caring for ourselves does not mean we have to check into the psychological unit of the hospital. It means taking care of what controls the rest of our bodies. Physical fitness is sluggish when the mind is sluggish. The mind is sluggish when encumbered with a load of worry, care and anxiety.

You may be mentally drained when you come home from work, when you go to bed and when you arise in the morning. Such constant mental drainage makes if difficult to improve your life. Therefore improving life demands mental rest. Allow your mind to take a break!

Every day we are faced with agendas, appointments, deadlines, school, homework, needs of kids, needs of parents, job pressures, dilemmas that need our attention. The list is endless. All of these and others can drain our minds. We react to the demands of life the following ways:

1. We worry. We worry about how we might change the scenario or add to it or take away from it. The trouble of worry is that it changes nothing. An old saying I've heard all my life is for every worry under the sun, either there is a cure or there is none. If there be one, seek till you find it, if there be none then never mind it.

   If you could worry about someone's sickness and make them better then you should stay up all night and worry. But truthfully it doesn't change anything.

2. We stress out. Stressing out is a deeper kind of worry. It is self-talk. It is becoming disoriented to reality. We are allowing the pressure to build to where we have no peace about anything going on in our lives. This can sometimes take the form of anxiety or even panic attacks.

    A panic attack is not pretty. It is when our dread, fear and stress level reaches a peak that may manifest itself in almost uncontrollable emotional behavior. We deal with it.

Here are some ways to deal with mental exhaustion.

1. Exercise. A family doctor said one time that the person who exercises in some form most every day would not need Prozac. I have no written support material to under gird that statement. Yet, in my own personal life I know for sure that when I exercise, the clouds and mental cobwebs seem to go away. A good two or three mile run or walk cleans out the system and seems to allow the body a chance to expel some toxins that otherwise could bring about harm to my body.

2. Rest. A rested mind is a sharper mind. There are days when you need to turn off the alarm clock. There are those days when the body is screaming, "Take a nap! I'm beat!" Listen to you body. If your foot is hurting it's trying to tell you something. If you are in need of rest, your body is telling you that it needs it. As we said previously you will feel more like exercising when you are rested. Plus, you will respond better to the different stresses and tensions that you will face throughout the day.

3. Make a reality assessment. We take careful stock of what
    is causing us to be so mentally exhausted. Is it because
    we are doing too much? Is it because we overestimate
    our importance? Have we plugged ourselves into so many
    committee meetings, projects, and extra work that we have
    spread ourselves too thin? When we spread ourselves
    into too many directions we will mentally try to give
    attention to every cause we have committed ourselves to.
    But the sheer thought of having to do so much can
    overwhelm us. You become mentally overwhelmed just
    thinking about it. Mental exhaustion can be the worst kind
    of tiredness.

4. Decide what is important. Before you can really pursue
    what is best you may have to give up what is good. I'm
    convinced many people are worn out doing good things
    and never get around to doing what is the very best for
    them. A wise friend said I don't have the time to do all the
    things that I want to do. Why would I ever want to
    try to do the things that I don't want to do?

    Every life will have duties and obligations that may not be
    exactly what we want to do at a certain time in our lives.
    There is no such thing as a life without obligation and total
    carefree living. Yet daily we must decide what we are going
    to give our minds and bodies to. Only we can make this
    mental decision. Once we've decided, then we feel a sense
    of rest about our lives. The mind is not pulled apart in ten
    directions. This brings us to point five.

5. Focus. A focused mind is a mind with a mission. You have
    decided what is important and now you are able to fully

concentrate. Even though you may have your daily ten-line to do list you know overall what you must be about for your life. Your ten-line to do list is those errands and activities that you will accomplish. But overall you understand what must be the priority. Jesus Christ was truly a focused man. He fed the hungry, healed the sick and taught his disciples. Yet, He knew His mission was even greater than these very important daily tasks. His mission was the overall redemption of mankind.

Fitness is a mind game. Mental exhaustion and cares that encumber you to the point of immobility are terribly unhealthy. Once you recognize that you are allowing worry and anxiety to stifle your life then you can move forward to handle these stresses and get your mind, body and life in shape!

Chapter 10

The Stagnate Life

You will find it harder to get into shape if you have allowed your life to become stagnate. I've heard more than once that if you want something done then ask a busy person to do it.

The life that is moving forward either mentally or physically indicates life. A life that has sat down and is motionless indicates death. Death can come in different forms.

1. There is a death of inactivity. Too often we see this in people who can't wait until they retire from a job. But then they spend the remaining days of their lives doing nothing. They feel they have earned the right to do nothing. Unfortunately doing nothing catches up with you. If you don't use your life you are going to lose it.

    The mind that is not used becomes dull. An active mind is a sharp mind. The muscles that are not used become limp and weak. An active body is a stronger body. If you don't read the newspaper or listen to the news you become out of touch with current events.

    The active life is a healthy life. It's possible to always do too much. Overload means imbalance. The back can carry only so much. The opposite is just as bad. When we have nothing to do we become imbalanced with under load.

    I recently drove through a city and was amazed at the

number of people I saw sitting in a section of the town on the street benches and leaning up against buildings. They weren't talking or doing anything. They just had this aimless look about them. It didn't look like a bus pickup place but a place where people came to do nothing. None of them looked very happy about what they were doing.

I can only imagine the following being said by too many in our world today: One of these days I'm going to retire. I'll do whatever I want, when I want. But the question is what will I want to do? Will I want to help, be productive, and make a difference; help somebody; pursue all those tasks that I never got to do? When I retire I will do what I want but what if I don't want to do anything…then what? The inactive life is like the Dead Sea. It takes water in but gives none out and therefore it is a dismal body of water.

2. The death of desire. When we lose the desire to do anything we have lost a major battle of life. We become stagnate because we don't want to do anything. You are closing in on death when there is no desire.

    I've seen many people on their deathbeds give up in those last couple of days. They are tired. They are weak. They have given in to total frustration. Nothing seems to be working right. The kidneys are shutting down, breathing is difficult, there may be tremendous discomfort, the body is not doing what you tell it to do and so desire to hang on gives way to the inevitable – death. What is it that keeps you going?

    How about you? Do you have a desire to live? Do you have

a desire to breathe? Do you have a desire to get out of bed in the morning? Do you have something to do? Do you have something to live for?

Too many lose the interest of living. Life is very much a mind game. The mind and life must have something to do. A daily plan of action is very important.

An old saying is that everyone needs something to do, someone to love and something to look forward to in order to have a life that feels complete. Jesus Christ is the answer to all three. He is someone to love. He has something for every life to do and He gives each of us something to look forward to daily and for eternity.

Christ also shapes the rest of our lives. He instills within us the desire to be productive. We know we have a purpose in life as long as we live and a part of our purpose is to take care of ourselves so that we can produce our very best. Loss of desire leads to inactivity and inactivity leads to a very unhealthy life.

Wrong Concept of Life

Somehow people have bought the concept that a wonderful life is one that achieves the freedom to do nothing.

The story is told of a train that had been going from the east coast to the west coast for many years and grew tired of going back and forth from one part of the country to the other. It dreamed of a day when it would no longer have to travel the track that kept it so bound. One day the train was going by a very beautiful meadow. The train thought to itself, that meadow is so lovely I think I want to go over there and just rest for a long time. The train managed to jump the track and into the meadow it sped. The meadow was truly lovely, but now the train was nothing but a wreck of piled up steel and metal. Never be useful again and never to move about freely from coast to coast.

Too many people have this understanding of life. Life, they believe, is achieving a time when one can sit down to never have to be mobile again if they do not wish to. Often people are like the train, one day they finally reach the meadow and it is gorgeous. But God did not make us to just totally jump the tracks of life. He made us to park beside the meadows. He made us to play in the meadows. He made us to appreciate the meadows. He made us to tend and cultivate the meadows. But, He did not make us to be useless in the meadow. People say, "I'm just going to jump in this flower garden and bask in the fragrance of the flowers." You can do that, but if you don't water it and pull the weeds the flower garden will lose its appeal.

There is little appeal to a stagnate life. The only thing you may say about a life that is stagnating is that all is the same. But not all is the same. Once life stagnates, it becomes dead and sad. The life that is stagnating says there is nothing to do. There is nothing that interests me. There is nothing that excites me. There are places to go but they do nothing for me.

What to Do

1. Pray for help. God will help you. He is strong. When you are weak and unable, He is very able.
2. Renounce idleness. This does not mean you renounce rest and sleep. The body, as we have already said, demands rest. Idleness is getting up from sleep to spend the entire day doing nothing. It's spending countless hours staring out

into space. It's sitting in the shade all day watching traffic go by. Again, every human being longs for a few days of life when we have the option to have such leisure time. Leisure moments are different than a daily lifestyle.

3.   Write down a few things that are important to you. What are they? Family? Other people? Someone? A school? A charity? Feeling better? Looking better? Someone may say I can think of nothing or nobody that is important to me. Nobody? Nothing? The world is big and there is much for us to be about doing. There are people to love. God has a purpose for every life.

4.   Make a mental commitment. Commit yourself to get your life going.
     The train that is off the track is the train that is going nowhere and has become only a heap of steel and nothingness. Make a decision that you are going to get on the track that leads to somewhere. Some swamps are hard to climb out of but you can. The Bible says, "I can do all things through Christ who strengthens me," Philippians 4:13. Make a mental decision to climb out of your rut. Anybody can get into a rut. You can run your car into a ditch. But you don't have to leave it there. Decide you are going to do whatever it takes to get out of your stagnate, boring state of life. Most often, your state of life happened because of the state of your mind. Change your attitude and you can change much of life about you.

5.   One day at a time. The only way you can accomplish your life is daily. You can plan for tomorrow but you live today until it comes. You can't go back and live yesterday. Yesterday has been lived. You can repent and apologize and even try to make restitution for any foul ups along the way. But you can't change yesterday. Too many today are

totally stagnated, immobilized, frozen by the past or the future. "Well, how did this happen? Why did that have to happen?" Or, "What is going to happen when this happens? What will become of us when such and such takes place." Often what has happened is that people have tried a few times and been beaten down and therefore have given up on life and are vegetating in stagnation. Or, they have worked so long they thought they would enjoy doing nothing but now realize it's not any fun but feel stuck in their aimlessness. Life is lived one day at a time.

6. Set achievable goals. Writing is big part of my life. I have learned about how much I can write every day. I can write two to six pages a day. There have been days when I have written ten pages. An average day for me is four or five pages five or six days a week. I seldom write on Sunday. I know that early in the day is the best time for me to write. I start writing between 4:00 – 5:00 in the morning and write to about 7:00. I can't write a book in a morning. I can't write a book in a week. When I look at a measly five pages and think about how big a project a book is, I wilt. But I know that if I write a little every day then my project will eventually be complete. If I only write one page a day I have 180 pages in six months. I know that I can write one page a day and I know that in time my project will be complete.

You can't lose 100 pounds in a week. It's possible that you can lose two pounds a week. It will require an effort. But that is something that you can do. The last twenty pounds or so will become a little more difficult but in one year's time your body weight can be radically reduced. Goals that are paced out over a longer period of time are far more easily reached.

Fitness is a mind game. Moving yourself out of immobility and stagnation requires one thing – a decision to do so. Decide right now to go forward with life. Ask God for power and strength. Ask Him for a mind to move forward.

Chapter 11

Conditions for Failure

We can be on the right path to physical and mental fitness but at the same time be immersed in unfavorable conditions. Regardless of our decisions to live and eat right we have to be very alert to our surroundings.

Surroundings can make or break us.

Your weight loss will face peril if these following conditions happen often in your weekly lifestyle.

1. **Buffets** – America has an increasing number of restaurants that offer all you can eat for a price. Many of these places are incredible opportunities to eat and eat and eat some more. For any person that has been trying to cut back and eat the right portions every day it can be a presentation of food that is difficult to turn down. One such place in my town is located conveniently close to my house. Within five minutes I can be at the buffet eyeing enough food to feed an army.

   Sure I can take two or three vegetables and a small portion of meat and salad and it could be a very nice meal. But the dessert island has everything and the food that I do eat is good. It's difficult to eat just one plate. One plate can easily become two or even three plates of food. The bread they bring to the table melts in your mouth. So how do you stop? It's tough.

   If you are seriously trying to lose weight you can't go to

buffets - at least not very often. Even if you only go once a week you can destroy all the hard work you have done in the previous six days. It's not worth undoing a week's worth of work in one hour.

Buffets are fast which makes them tempting. We live in a fast paced, hurry up society. A person can pull the car into the parking lot, run in and chomp down 3000 calories real quick. How long will it take to shed that meal? It will take far longer to shed it than it did to add it to your body.

Fitness requires thought. Fitness is a mind game. You determine the day before, or at the beginning of your day how you are going to do your best to live as right as possible for that day.   Then you go through that day. At the end of the day you rejoice over your victories for the day. You rejoice that you were able to eat sensible healthy portions of food that did not add up to more than what your daily allotment is. You celebrate the exercise that you did whether it was twenty minutes or an hour. You rejoice over the projects that were begun or even completed. You give thanks for all the good people that you were associated with for the day and the opportunities to love and to be loved. These are all blessings that you give thanks and praise for. Then you go to sleep and rest because you are likely tired. In the morning you are ready, once again, to have another good day.

Success in weight loss and life fitness is stacking up the good days. One commercial advertises their product and says, "Give us a week and we'll take off the weight." That is probably true. Do anything regimented for seven days and you will see results. Seven days of regimented, calculated eating. Each day you think about what you are going to eat and how you are going to do life. You are making decisions about your life and body.

The buffet chow trough is allowing an obstacle to appear in your path of right living that you don't need. Of course, I am not saying that you can never go to one of these restaurants. I am saying you are likely setting yourself up for a setback that may be discouraging to you when you step on the scale the next morning.

Consider the next peril of disaster to weight reduction.

2. **Full Refrigerators** – The average American feels impoverished if there is not enough food in the refrigerator to feed five families. But what happens when you have extra snacks, and quick food items available in your refrigerator? You eat them.

    One battle I fight if I am home and have any time at all on my hands, is standing in front of the refrigerator with the door open. I don't know what I am expecting to appear or disappear since I last looked. And, if there is an assortment of ice cream sandwiches, candy bars or cold cut meats available I'm likely to indulge.

    The person on the path to fitness must stock the refrigerator very carefully. Don't buy all that extra stuff at the store. Think about the obvious. Who is going to eat this food you are buying? Chances are, even if you have kids, you are likely to eat your share. If you do the grocery shopping you probably buy the kinds of snacks that you like. And, if you like them then you are putting a daily temptation right in front of your eyes every time you open the refrigerator door.

Stock your refrigerator with only what you need to make your week successful. Consider bottled water to replace sugar filled soft drinks. All kinds of nutritional fitness bars are on the market. Look for ones with low sugar content. Some nutritional candy bars are no better than a regular chocolate bar. So, learn to read the backside for content.

Most importantly find something to do other than gaze into your refrigerator. Life is more than standing in front of the refrigerator. If it doesn't have a lot of extra stuff in it, then you are not likely to battle going back and forth grabbing snacks and undoing any fitness plan that you are on.

3.   Avoid people who live only to eat. This may sound cruel. But we live in a culture where the only outlet people have is eating. They eat for recreation, they eat for love, they eat as a hobby, and they eat when there is a lot to do or when there is nothing to do. Many of these good intentioned people what to share their lives with you. They want to share their recreation and they want to share their love with you. Eating with somebody can be a very pleasant experience. But when the experience becomes, "Why aren't you eating more? How come you are not having dessert? Why won't you eat more bread?" Then the experience becomes less than enjoyable for the person who may be in daily battle to shed some weight. It becomes more of a trial and a hardship.

The well intended person thinks they are being a good host for pushing another helping. I have even been with people who became irritated with me because I would not eat more. I couldn't help it they had made enough for ten people! I am only one person!

An offer to eat more is the gracious thing for the host to do. A reply from the guest who says, "No thanks, I am full." should be enough.

Eating should be a delightful experience that adds to the fulfillment of our lives and not to the downfall of our lives. There can be nothing better than sitting down with family or friends and sharing food. Some of the greatest experiences in the Bible took place around food. Jesus ate the last supper with his disciples. It was an incredible experience of fellowship and intimate conversation. When He sat in the house of the tax collector it was at a meal. It was during this meal that Zacchaeus, a very wealthy man determined he would change his life and begin to be what God wanted him to be and help others who were less fortunate. In the wilderness God gave to Moses and his people what they needed to eat every day. Each day what they needed was provided.

Fitness is a mind game. When you go to the table with friends or family use good sense in what and how much you eat. Remember, you have a plan. Your plan may allow you to eat anywhere from 200, 600 or maybe even 700 calories. Make the experience one that, when you leave the table, you feel good about what has happened and not set back by what has happened. Make the meal an experience

that advances your life for the better and not one that
debilitates it for the worse.

4. **Debilitating People** – These are the people who always find
    a way to negate your eating and exercise habits. Normally
    these are people who know they need to lose weight and
    have not made the mental decision to do it. Often it is not
    until the doctor demands that they gain control of their
    eating patterns that they start making an effort to eat more
    selectively.

These people will plant words into your mind like, "You
look great." It's nice to hear that when you know you look
great. But, when you know that you couldn't fasten your
dress or trousers on that day, things are not right. The
last thing you need to hear is somebody trying to flatter
you when you know that you are desperate to lose twenty
pounds. Most of us know when we look the best that we
can possibly look. We know when we are our best. We
also know when we are fair or not so great. We know it by
how we feel. We know by how our clothes feel on us. We
know by our energy level. We know when we look into
the mirror. The last thing we need is somebody telling us
something that we know is not true.

Avoid people who put you down for exercising. People may
joke with you about your exercising patterns but if you are
constantly rubbing shoulders with someone who is putting
you down for your exercise efforts and it is affecting your
efforts then you need to distance yourself from this person.

Fitness is a mind game. You do not need to hear negative

stuff about what you are trying to do. You are truly in a battle for life. Why open your life to daily criticism?

5. **Other Social Situations.** People gather around food. Civic groups, political groups, church groups and gatherings of friends and families always have food. Have fun and watch the landmines. Such social gatherings present conditions for failure on your path to weight loss and life fitness.

The landmines are those great looking dishes of food and desserts that you never intended to allow yourself to come upon. You just walk through the line and bang they are there. You take a big spoon full of this and a big spoon full of that. Soon, you have a plate that is going to go down so wonderfully good. But, it will all be there for you to see on the scale the very next day. Walk circumspectly at these social occasions. Before you go, make a mental note what you are going to face. It will look and taste good. But will it be good for you the next day? Will you feel good about yourself the next morning?

When I attended the rotary we always ate at the best restaurant in town with the best buffet. It was so good. Any church that I have ever been affiliated with has always had the best cooks in the world. I have never been a part of a church where the women could not cook and bake incredible food. I know that at any Wednesday night meal at my church where the ladies are responsible for cooking, I can easily gain two pounds.

Fitness involves mental awareness of the conditions that could set us back or detour us on our path to success.

Chapter 12

Conditions for Success

A garden produces a good crop under the right conditions.

First, the field must be prepared. The ground must be tilled and then fertilized.

Second, seed is sown.

Third, water and sunshine and time produce visible signs of the farmer's success.

Fourth, there must be cultivation of the crop. Weeds are pulled that might smother the harvest. The crop is inspected often for any bugs or insects that might be detrimental to the full maturity of the crop.

Fifth, the harvest is collected.

Sixth, the harvest is enjoyed!

It's important to note that at any time the crop can be destroyed or severely crippled. Poor preparation, improper seeding, insufficient water and neglectful watch care of the crop can only produce poor results. The farmer wants good results! Why waste your time producing a bad garden?

You can bring about fitness to your body but you need to create and allow the conditions for success.

1. Buy a smaller pair of jeans. If you wear a waist size 38 then buy a waist size 36. If you are a lady do the same. Buy a pair of jeans that you are too big for and start working to fit into them. Pick out one day a week to try them on. Some days you won't have the heart to try them on because you know there is no way they are going to fit. But make yourself do it and it will be a mental stimulator to you. The stimulation

will be that reminder that you still have work to do.

2.   Buy a set of scales. There are different theories about scales. Some people believe that you should never step on a scale. However for me, scales draw me back to the track. If I have been eating poorly it will show in how my jeans feel. But the scale numbers will also tell the truth. Make sure your scales are right. A good set will tell you how you have done over the previous seven days. Weigh yourself at about the same time once a week.

3.   Associate with some fitness people. People who start fitness/ weight loss programs are more successful if they have a few friends who are like-minded. It's vital that you meet with these people every week or two. These may be people that you actually work out or run with.

There are runner's clubs that will welcome you. This group will meet at least once a week to do a three, five or ten mile run. If you are not this visionary yet, then go to someplace where others are walking and running. The setting or environment will be an encouragement to you to do likewise. This is where health clubs and gyms help. In such an environment you will be around others trying to accomplish many of the same goals that you are.

4.   Find a workout buddy. This may be a person that you jog or run with or someone that you meet at the gym to lift weights. At the outset, it could be someone to just talk with about weight loss and eating ideas. For a person starting out fitness, routine reading and studying the right books may be the very start of their process. However, having

someone else to compare notes and thoughts with is a plus.
A routine buddy provides the following benefits:

    a.   You have somebody to work out with you.

    b.   Workouts are often easier when you have somebody else to work with you.

    c.   Buddies will keep each other working out. There is the certainty that next week is coming and each of you are responsible for making sure the other is going to show up for exercise.

    d.   Buddies are to encourage each other about eating right and staying true to a fitness lifestyle until the next appointed time.

5.   Set a goal. A goal that is not visualized is a goal that is not attained. The archer aims for the bull's eye. The builder has drawings that he is building toward. His blueprints keep him on track. They are the goal. Without a vision you will not make it. Your vision is what you are going to become. Your vision is how you are going to look. Your vision includes how great you are going to feel!

Just as a farmer envisions his crop you are envisioning your success. It could take you a year to achieve your program. But what if you don't set a goal. Then where are you going to be a year from now? Are you going to be twenty pounds heavier than you are today? Goals not set are goals not attained. Write down exactly how much weight you want to lose. Write down exactly what clothes size you want to attain. Write down your other goals. Maybe it's to run a five-mile race. Maybe it's to reach a certain level of tennis ability or other activity. Life either goes forward or backward. If you are not going forward you begin to stagnate, dry up and die.

6. Use it. Use your body. If you don't, you'll lose it. The
    longer you let your garden go without any cultivation
    the harder it is to rescue it and bring it back to shape. It
    works the same way with the body. Tie your arm to your
    side long enough and it will soon need therapy to bring it
    back to use. God gave you a body. Use it. Work it. Hard
    work doesn't hurt people. Sweating does not hurt you. God
    made your body in such a way that it could release many of
    the toxins and poisons that threaten your health. A good
    sweat releases these and cleans your body. When the heart
    rate is elevated and the sweat begins to flow then you are
    giving your body a release that it well deserves.

    But if you don't work or exercise your body then you are
    going to miss this necessity for life fitness. God made
    Adam to till and care for the garden that He had placed
    him in. His work would be a sense of fulfillment for him.
    The youngest acting and looking senior adults that I know
    are seniors who continue to work and play way past their
    65th birthday. Two of my dear friends who are 80 years
    old work all the time. My father now 82 at this writing is
    active every day mowing grass, using his trimmer around
    the house and walking hills. My mother made it to 85.
    She battled Alzheimer's and mini strokes. However, when
    she was 82, she was pushing the lawn mower a couple
    of days a week. The next summer she decided to quit
    pushing the lawn mower. She became inactive and her
    health went down like a rock. I can't say that, with her
    disease of Alzheimer's, she would not have dropped any
    way. However, I find in so many instances that seniors and

people who stay physically active seem to stay younger longer. They do not retire to sedentary lives. Even after retiring from a job or vocation they find ways to keep their bodies active.

7.   Read the Bible. I know of no other book that promotes physical and mental fitness more than the Bible. The Bible says our bodies are the temple of God. The Spirit of God dwells in each believer. Why would we want to neglect or abuse where God dwells?

The Bible tells us about a man who was filled with demons. His life was such a wreck that he lived among tombs and afflicted pain to his body. Those who lived nearby could hear his wails of pain and it was scary for them as they heard this man. The Bible tells us how Jesus delivered him from the legion of evil that lived within him and enabled him to regain his right mind. When he regained his right frame of mind he quit abusing his body and was at peace with himself. When Job lost his health he sat in misery. Could it be that after he lost all his children and money that he mentally grieved himself into his illness? Loss of relationships and financial security can be mentally and therefore physically debilitating if we allow it to.

Have you ever seen a fat Jesus? I've never seen an artist rendition of a fat Jesus. I hear so many Christian people talk about following Jesus, then eat like pigs and almost refuse to exercise. None of us want to hang on a cross. Jesus did that for us. But if He truly looked as artists have painted him over the years then he was one lean, good-looking man. I don't think Mary and Martha were sexually attracted to Jesus. Jesus was pure and holy and that was what attracted these women to Christ. It was the same qualities that attracted the other disciples to Jesus. He was the genuine Son of God. However, could Jesus have attracted His disciples and people like Mary and Martha and others had he been a fat slob who sat around eating everything in sight?

Jesus was a carpenter. He worked with his hands. It was a good form of physical and mental fitness. He walked a lot. People in this day didn't have many choices of transportation. If they went somewhere they had to pack up and take off walking. All of this walking, along with hard work, made them very physically fit.

Jesus also took care of his mental attitude. Time and again, throughout the scriptures, we read about Jesus going to a mountain to pray. Or, he would separate himself from the throngs of people, for a period of time, to spend time with the Father. It helped him to face the tasks of the day.

God made you and there will never be anybody else like you. That doesn't mean that we can't improve or be better. If we don't strive in life then we would never go to school. We would just say this is the level of intelligence that I have. This is what I was born with and therefore I'll just accept what God has given to me. We could say this about everything. It is a true blessing to live with a level of contentment. If we can't ever find any contentment then we are miserable, restless people. But the contentment comes after the work. The garden is enjoyed after it brings forth the fruit. There is joy in cultivating it. We find peace in knowing that we are doing the right thing in taking care of it. If we let it go to waste then we look at it and see only failure, that makes us feel bad. However, success makes us feel great.

Weight loss and fitness encourages us. We are unique and God gave us minds to use. We take care of ourselves to the best of our ability. Therefore, we feel good about who we are because we are being a good caretaker of the body that God gave to us.

Chapter 13

Ideas that Work

Fitness is a great way to think and live. The goal of a fit body and mind complement each other to make the best of daily life.

Fitness is not drudgery. The idea of making your body the best possible, is not a burden, it's a delight! Fitness is about you. Most of us spend our lives working for others and caring for others but your program of fitness is about your body and life. And when you take care of you, then you will do a better job of taking care of people you love. You will be a better worker at whatever your job is in life.

We make exercise drudgery. We dread walking or running the miles. We dread the abdominal exercises. We dread working our muscles. Why? We don't dread feeding our faces. We don't dread eating 1500 calories at a single meal and adding on fat – at least we don't until we look in the mirror or our clothes won't fit! Pushing the lawn mower, taking a swim or walking eighteen holes of golf is something good that you are doing for the body that God gave to you.

The hardest part of walking or running is putting your shoes on and walking out the door. It means making a move in the right direction. When you are finished you are tired and sweating but your body loves it. You have done something to release some of the pent up tension and poisons that are plugging up your body and making it inefficient. The arteries in your heart thank you for burning off some of the fat and cholesterol that makes its purpose harder. Your muscles thank you for giving them the chance to be used.

Ideas that Work

1. **Walking** – Start out with a goal of two miles and you may
    build up to three or more as needed. You determine if you
    need more. It's okay to walk five miles if that's all you are
    doing. But you need a balanced exercise program and it's
    not in your best interest to just walk. But, walking is great.
    If you have one or two other people to walk with this can
    be a great social outing. You will pass the time quickly if
    you have someone interesting to talk to along the way. Or,
    invest in a small radio that you can strap on or carry in your
    pocket. Just don't turn it up so loud that you are oblivious
    to traffic and your surroundings. If you are walking on a
    sidewalk it's not as dangerous as a road, yet you need to be
    aware of what is happening around you. Carrying a disc or
    cassette player gives you the opportunity to listen to some
    of your favorite music. Upbeat music that makes you move
    a little faster is the best kind.

    Walk in pretty weather or walk in the rain. Some of the
    best walks I've had have been on rainy days. You can buy a
    light hooded jacket to keep you semi dry. The world looks
    different on a rainy day and you will be amazed at all the
    problems in your life you can work through on a rainy day
    walk. Of course stay in the house if it's thundering and
    lightning. Always use common sense.

    Walking is good for any time of the day. Early morning or
    evening walks or the middle of the day; there is no bad
    time for a good walk unless it is dangerously hot. Make your
    walk a time that is good for you. Make it a fun time. Early
    morning or lunchtime may be the best. If you walk after

eight at night be warned that it could make you stay up later. The body has to wind down and slow down in order to hit the bed and go to sleep.

Another tip for walkers is changing the places you walk. Make walking an adventure or like a new trip you are taking. You will see new sights along your journey.

A comfortable pair of shoes is vital. If your feet are hurting then you are not going to have fun. Save your money and buy a new pair of shoes every six months – at least. Some heavy runners buy a new pair of shoes every three months. Listen to your feet they will tell you when they are hurting. Often, it's because of the shoes you are wearing.

2. **Home Exercise** – Many people exercise in their homes. You may have a treadmill or something else that you use. You may exercise while watching your favorite movie or listening to your favorite CD. For you the privacy of your home and own entertainment may be what does it for you. I do not have a gym in my home. I live in a 2200 square foot house and I don't have the space for exercise equipment.

However, I do have a garage. I use my garage to park two cars and then there are the many boxes that have junk in them. I am clueless as to what is in these boxes. Someday, I will find out! The garage is a great place to exercise. I can jump rope do jumping jacks and push-ups. I can even turn on the battery to one of the cars and listen to a radio station or play a CD while exercising. This works especially well in cold winter weather. Sit-ups can be done in your house on a rug or your carpet. You can finish up the morning news while you do your ten or fifty abdominal crunches. Creativity always keeps exercise stimulating and fun. You won't want to do garage exercise every day. After a few weeks it's boring. But it's okay occasionally for something different. Exercise requires periodically changing your pattern to keep yourself interested and motivated.

3. **Running** – Yes walking and running are two different spectrums. Running is far more intense. Running pushes the body and the heart muscle and truly delivers some amazing results. Faithful runners will have sleek, trim healthy bodies, if they are careful of what they eat! Any exercise program can undo itself quicker than it can help by camping out in front of the refrigerator after the three-mile run is over. Keep in mind if you run three miles that you may burn off 500 calories or a little more. But one Big Mac sandwich will put 600 calories and mega fat grams right back into your body. That kind of life is not fun. You have wasted your important, precious time when you treat your body that way.

    Running is something that you can leave your house and do fast. You can have it done and over with in 30 minutes. A good 30-minute run burns the fat, is fast and revitalizes your spirit. You don't have to jump in your car and drive twenty minutes to get to your workout spot. You can run around your subdivision or the road where you live. During your run you have time to think, laugh, cry, pray or let out whatever is inside of you. Or, you can take in the beauty of the world that God has made.

A running buddy helps. Running is more difficult when you have someone you have to meet at a certain time. It makes the process longer as far as getting the workout over. But from a fun perspective it really helps some days to have someone to push you a little. There will be many days when you will want to utilize your running time as a time for you to think and clear out some of your mental challenges or cobwebs.

4. **Weight Lifting** – Few people systematically lift weights. But careful weight lifting is vital for life fitness. I'm not talking about bodybuilding. Body builders work for a very defined, carved look. Sometimes that look may be very bulky or a smaller leaner look. The average person thinks that if they start lifting some weights that they are ultimately trying to look like someone posed on a muscle magazine. That kind of look requires a total commitment of one's life and energy. And it is not a look that is for everybody. Frankly only a few people really want to look that way. For those who do it's fun and good – so be it. Most people aren't really into massive muscle building. They want to lose weight, look better in their clothes, feel good and be as healthy as they can possibly be. These are truly worthy goals. Weight lifting is helpful in this process.

Weight lifting builds a body that burns the fat. A fat, limp body stores more fat. Muscle weighs more than fat, but it burns fat away and gives you a leaner healthier look and feeling. Weight lifting may sound like drudgery. It can be. But use weights that you are comfortable lifting. Don't try to go to a gym and break records. You may at first want to exercise on five or ten pounds for biceps and three pounds for triceps. You will be amazed what repetition will do for you even though you are using light weights. Find a buddy to lift with. It's more fun and motivating when someone else is encouraging you.

5. **Tennis** – This sport is rigorous and takes practice. But with tennis you need someone to play with which makes it a great social hour. You will be amazed at the camaraderie you will develop and experience as you meet new tennis partners. Plus you will have a fun workout. Keep in mind that it's about your body and fitness experience. Your goal is to sweat and exercise your body. But having fun and being with nice people are extra-added qualities.

6. **Swimming** – In most places swimming is a seasonal activity unless you have access to an indoor pool. If you do, it can be a wonderful way to treat your body. There is no stress on the feet and knees and you are receiving an overall workout. The heart rate can be greatly accelerated. Try a twenty-minute swim of laps up and down the pool and you will be one tired person when it's over.

7. **Bicycling** – There is nothing like riding a bike for three or four miles. It's truly an aerobic workout. This is why many health clubs today now offer classes called "Spinning." Spinning is riding a stationary exercise bike for 45 minutes to an hour. The levels of tension can be increased or decreased to simulate changing gears on a ten-speed bike or going up and down hills. The class is done with a group of people and to upbeat music, which makes it fun and energizing.

8. **Aerobics** – Aerobics might be considered any kind of motion with the body that elevates the heartbeat for a long

enough time period to burn some calories and some fat. I do
aerobics a lot. Well, at least one class or two classes a week.
Some weeks I do more. But normally I try to mix in two
hard pumping aerobic classes a week. I usually do about 30
to 45 minutes of the class. Most people do the whole hour
or more. Everybody is different. I personally enjoy doing
the abdominal exercises in the gym. But many like doing
the stomach exercises under the direction of the instructor.
Whatever works for you is best.

Aerobics are done as free floor movements, on steps and
even with weights. They are all effective and you will get
out of the class whatever you put into it. I often turn it up a
notch and work very hard in these classes. Aerobic classes
provide you with an instructor who guides you in motions
you can make to elevate your heartbeat. However, it's
very easy to lay back in a class and just barely go through
the motions and never break a sweat. Or, you can work
hard and walk out of the class, soaking wet with sweat as I
normally do. There have been some classes that I finished
where I barely had a dry spot left on my shirt. That is when
I feel I really had a workout!

9. **Hiking** – Some of the best exercise can be walking hills
    and mountain paths. A hike is more of an event. You may
    begin in the early morning and spend the day walking,
    climbing and surveying the very beauty of God's outdoors.
    Pack water and some nutritious snacks. A good hike could
    involve several miles and burn off one bunch of calories!

10. **White Water Rafting** – This is the kind of exercise that is
    not readily available for the average person. Most people

have to drive to where the action is happening. Rafting trips can last as briefly as an hour and as long as four hours and even more. You paddle at times with intensity on some of these excursions and when the trip is over you have had one very nice workout – plus a blast of fun! This kind of experience may not be an instant blast of aerobic activity. However, when you are doing something recreational plus staying away from the meal table at the same time it has positive benefits.

11. **Rock Climbing** – This sport is not for everybody. But, I am told that what it does to your arm and leg muscles over the course of a couple of hours of climbing is incredible. For those who love sailing off the high cliffs with a safety rope it truly must be an exhilarating experience. But, I'll pass on that one.

12. **Golf** – This can be a good workout if you want it to be. If you walk and pull your cart you can truly burn off some real calories. If you play eighteen holes and drink water you are doing yourself some good. Even if you must ride a cart it's a fun way to be outdoors and still burn off a few calories. However, if you ride along in your cart eating junk food you are only kidding yourself that you are doing something fit.

13. **Bowling** – Bowling doesn't look like much of a workout. But, just try one night of it. Try rolling that ball down a lane for two or three games and see how you feel the next morning. Remember your proper form! Use your legs, back and arms correctly and you will know that you used some different muscles when you awaken the next morning!

14. **Lawn Mowing** – I honestly dread mowing the yard. It's so weird that I can run two or three miles and go to the gym and lift weights but wilt when I look at my tiny yard! It's simply dreading something that's boring to me. A radio headset helps. Watch your hearing on this one though. Don't crank up the volume to where you are drowning out the sound of your mower. Some upbeat music or a good inspirational tape will make the time fly by. If I have something good to listen to I can make that grass disappear faster.

15. **Housecleaning** – Picking up dirty clothes, dusting and doing any kind of housework can be a mundane tedious same old kind of thing. Look at it this way – when you are cleaning house you are on your feet doing something. Likely you are not eating because you are busy. If you are in motion and not nibbling on food then you are doing something positive that is going to give you a good feeling when it is over. You won't burn a bunch of calories or fat. But if it takes you a couple of hours to put your house into order then it might surprise you how many calories you have burned. The constant motion of using your legs and arms could easily burn off three or four hundred calories in a couple of hours. I only burn off four hundred calories when I go with all my might for twenty minutes on a stair master machine at the gym. While the house cleaning calories take longer, you still accomplish some calorie burn plus get your house in order!

16. **Wash and Wax Your Car** – Car washes are so prevalent today. But if you want a good work out then get the bucket of soapy water, rag and water hose out and wash your car. Dry it and apply the wax. The movement of waxing your

car and then removing the wax will give your arms and upper body one very good tedious work out! Plus, you will have one good-looking car!

17. **Learn To Play** – Didn't you play when you were a child? When I was a kid I loved playing hide and seek and tag and other games with community kids. We shot basketball, played baseball, kickball, swam and rode our bicycles and laughed and just had fun. My childhood experience of playing a lot kept me very lean. When I was 14, I was 6'1 and weighed 135 pounds. Yes…I was skinny! And when I was 18, I was 6'3 and weighed 185 pounds. I played basketball all the time, ran the mile in 5 minutes and 30 seconds, and was one athletic guy – and life was fun. Everything I did was fun. Also…put basketball in the line up of activities. At this very time I occasionally play with a 67 year old man who beats me one on one as much as I beat him. He looks great.

It's so tragic that we quit playing. We graduate from school and of course we have to work to make our way and then we marry and have kids and life can become very tedious and daily. We look forward to becoming adults and then one day we are adults and then we start acting like adults - old dried up ones! If I did not do aerobic exercise classes, run, and lift weights I think I would lose my mind. For twelve years my wife daily declined with multiple sclerosis. For five years I cared for her like a baby. She became a total invalid before she died. Enough said about that, "Silent Struggler" is my book about being a caregiver and "Nursing Home Nightmares" tells about that segment of our lives.

If I refused to allow myself to do anything fun then life would have been over for me. The stress would build to such a level that my heart would explode and then I would be in heaven. Of course, heaven will be an awesome place but I don't think God wants us to push our way there. There is enough toil, strife, unpleasant circumstances, sickness and misery that life will try to hand to us every day. If there is any way we can have some fun kinds of exercise excursions then go for it! Hey, when it comes to fun…it doesn't even have to be exercise! But if you can do something that's healthy for the body that makes you smile and even laugh then that is the best of both worlds.

18. **On and On** – There is so much you can do. Volleyball is one great exercise. Fencing is an incredible workout. I took a semester of fencing (sword fighting), at Georgetown College and when I removed the facemask I was burning up with sweat. Plus it's fun. Horseshoes is fun. Throwing the baseball or shooting hoops in the driveway are fun. The main thing is doing something besides lying on the couch and clicking the television remote. About all you are getting out of that is exercising one poor little finger! Plus you are probably munching on snacks and becoming a large couch potato! After awhile you have put on weight. You don't laugh anymore. You don't even smile. You feel bad about yourself. You feel sorry for yourself. You hate how you can't get into your clothes anymore. You probably are not easy to live with. Because you feel bad about yourself then you are likely difficult to live with. You say things you don't mean to say. You act pitiful and you hate being that way. So…stop it. Change your life!

Fitness is a mind game! Just make up your mind that you are going to trim down, lose weight and you are going to laugh every day! You are especially going to laugh when you step on that scale every week and see the pounds rolling away!

Chapter 14

Laugh with People
Don't make fun of them!

The reason so many people fear exercise is because it's such a break from what they normally do. Normalcy to the average person is getting up, cleaning up and going to work and then coming home and mowing the grass, taking a shower and going to bed. Or, going through other basic routines of life.

The idea of exercising to so many is scary because if they go walking or running around the subdivision or down the road somebody might see them! The idea of being seen and fearing that somebody might snicker about us in our walking or jogging attire is completely unnerving to many would be exercisers.

Have you ever looked at a walker and thought, "That person really needs to be walking." However, you respected them for being out trying to do something positive.

We fear going to a track to walk because that's something we haven't done before and it's new uncharted territory. We fear going to a gym because we are clueless about what to do with all those machines, gadgets and weights! Plus, we know there are some awesome looking people in those gyms and so there is insecurity that keeps many of them from even making an appearance at a gym.

There is silliness about anything we do until it becomes so customary that it's routine to us. I felt silly the first time I played tennis. I could not hit that ball! When I did it went clear over the fence! I know people probably chuckled at me swatting at the tennis ball. To this day I am not much of a golfer. Believe me I am very paranoid when I tee off in front of a group of people. Most of the time people are nice but I can just feel that someone is dying to chuckle a little when I swing one or two times and miss the entire ball! But I swallow my pride and play any way. You can't learn to hit the ball if you never swing at it! Unfortunately, it's just taking me a while longer than it seems to take other people. I go to church with some excellent bowlers who can royally thrash me when it comes to bowling.

Don't ever look at people who are trying to exercise and say they look silly or stupid. They may look silly and people can be really funny. Laugh with them but don't laugh at them.

I bet Michael Jordan looked funny the first time he played basketball. Did anybody ever laugh at him in College or the NBA? No…he played with the greatest of ease and he was something to behold. What about the tennis champions and ice-skating champions of the world? We sit and watch them in a state of wonder. There was probably a time that they looked a little silly starting out. No one begins as a champion. Everybody begins at the starting place.

Lifting weights or using the machines at a gym may seem weird to you. You feel like your self consciousness could not handle it and therefore you shrink back from even trying. Fitness is a mind game. There are those moments when you mentally have to win out and overcome yourself and say, "I can do it! With God's help… I can do it!"

Aerobic exercise can truly look real stupid. I'm sure that anybody seeing a class for the first time would say, "Those people are stupid acting." But what looks stupid produces an incredible workout.

When you decide to get into shape you have to decide that you are going to swallow your pride. You buy a comfortable pair of shoes, shorts, athletic socks and a tee shirt and get with it.

You can begin at home doing simple exercises before you move outdoors to pursue all the possibilities of fitness that lie outside. The main thing is to start.

You were excited about driving a car. But you may have been a little apprehensive about the first day you got under the wheel. You knew you could pull it off, but you may have questioned yourself a little. When you learned to ride a bicycle or swim there were those early beginnings when it seemed tough, then suddenly you got the hang of it and there was no turning back.

Starting a fitness program of proper eating and exercise is much the same way. You begin and know that once you're into it, the inferiority feeling goes away and there is no turning back!

Chapter 15

Attitude

Attitude will make you or break you. Exercise and life fitness is not so hard…it's our attitude about it. If you take the attitude that something is impossible it will be. If you believe you can't walk or run three miles then you won't.

When you say, "I can't," then you won't. If you look in the mirror and say there is no way I can have the body that I really want, then guess what? You won't.

Being a caregiver to a sick wife can be really hard. Or, it can be different. I chose to accept the philosophy that it was different. Because something is different does not make it all that hard. It's my attitude about the difference that determines how hard it is.

Any job can start out hard but the test of enduring any job is our willingness to stick it out and learn the secrets to making it easy. Jobs begin hard because we are in a wilderness land. We don't know the geography. We don't know where the bumps are and when we accidentally stumble over them they hurt and stress us out. But when we know where they are then we can easily step around or over them or know exactly how to fall the right way when we trip again! The attitude to tackling any new assignment must be one of taking one day at a time and slowly learning the process.

The right thinking will make you and the wrong thinking will break you.

The world is filled with so much wrong thinking.

As a person thinks in his heart so is he.

A good attitude and a fit mind work together.

A fit mind finds its joy in the Lord.

From the Bible Philippians 4:4 says, "Rejoice in the Lord always, I will say it again: Rejoice! Attitude comes when you don't find your happiness in circumstances. Circumstances change. If you find your joy in a sunny day then your joy will change often because not every day in life is sunny. If you find your happiness in things then you'll never be permanently happy because things wear out, breakdown or are passed on to somebody else. Find your joy in the Lord, He never changes. Jesus said, in John 15:11, "I have told you this so that my joy may be in you and that your joy may be complete." Psalm 16:11 says, "You have made me with joy in your presence, with eternal pleasures at your right hand." A right attitude knows that God is for us. We don't always like the circumstances. Circumstances can be challenging. Fifty pounds to lose can be a daunting trial. Your attitude must be that this is not impossible and your circumstances can change for the better and not the worse. Your joy is in God and He will see you through.

Next, Attitude is complemented when we know God is with us. Paul says in Philippians 4: 5, "Let your gentleness be evident to all, the Lord is near." You are not alone in whatever you face. God is with you. Attitude takes hold of whatever adversity there is in life and says I can deal with this adversity because God is with me. I don't have to handle this alone.

Attitude does not live in the worry zone. Worry is an awful state of mind and a terrible place to live. In verse six of this scripture Paul says, "Do not be anxious about anything, but in everything, by prayer and petition, with thanksgiving, present your requests to God."

Worry in the Greek language means to divide. Worry means we are pulled apart in our lives. Worry clouds our attitude. It's difficult to believe in ourselves and feel we can overcome the situation if we are worried sick about something.

Jesus warned against worry in Matthew 6:27, "Who of you by worrying can add a single hour to his life?" A little saying that I've heard all my life is, for every worry under the sun, either there is a cure or there is none. If there be one, seek till you find it, if there be none, never mind it. You cannot lose one pound by worry. You cannot add one dollar to your pocket by worry. Yet, all around us in our world people are stressed to the max with worry.

For a great attitude boost – try prayer. The scripture says in verse 6, "Do no not be anxious about anything, but in everything, by prayer and petition, with thanksgiving, present your requests to God." We should learn to pray about everything. There is nothing about our lives that is too big or too small for God. Is there anything about your life that is big for God? God is bigger than all of our problems. Try taking them to Him in prayer.

A great attitude is a thankful attitude. When you learn to thank God in all things that is the highest expression of faith.

How can we be thankful for multiple sclerosis, cancer, Alzheimer's, unemployment, debilitation and even an extra 50 pounds to lose? Romans 8:28 says, "All things work together for good to them who love God." This does not mean we always understand. It does not mean that we do not get pressed down, perplexed and confused. It does not mean that we are people without emotions. It does not mean that we do not pray for help or healing or for miracles. But we do it with the attitude that we can make strides in our lives regardless of the situation. Often, the greatest stride we have to make is in the mind.

Positive thinking is a must! Even the scripture teaches positive thinking. In verse 8 we read, "Whatever is true, whatever is noble, whatever is right, whatever is pure, whatever is lovely, whatever is admirable – if anything is excellent or praiseworthy-think about such things."

Our minds control our actions. Sow a thought – reap an act. Sow an act reap a habit.

The Bible tells us to think about what is right and what is

lovely. Is sitting on the sofa devouring a bag of chips, a candy bar and two soft drinks lovely? It might be okay once every three months…but not every day. Think about what is lovely. Think about what you can become. Think about how far you can go with your life. You are limited only by wrong, negative thinking.

I suggest you have a thirty-minute to one-hour quiet time with God every morning. Use the time to focus on what you and God need to accomplish for the day. You may zero in on one or two verses from the Bible. Write down what you would like to accomplish for the day. Your goals for eating and exercise are a part of this quiet time. Write down what you will allow yourself to eat and what your exercise goals are for the day. This requires some discipline, but will show a great pay off when you step on the scales.

Stay busy. The scripture says in verse nine, "Whatever you have learned or received or heard from me, or seen in me – put it into practice. And the God of peace will be with you."

Busyness is not an end in itself. We do not work to make ourselves acceptable to God. God makes us acceptable to Him by His grace.

Verse seven is my favorite in this passage, "And the peace of God, which transcends all understanding, will guard your hearts and minds in Christ Jesus."

There is nothing better than a heart and a mind that is at peace. When we are at peace about our lives we are free to run, jump, laugh, play, eat healthy and celebrate every moment of every day because we know that with God's help we can deal with whatever has come our way and work through the situation to soar above the circumstance.

Chapter 16

Unhealthy Thinking

There are four very unhealthy emotions that can be detrimental to your pursuit of life fitness. They may even make you more prone to eat food that you really don't need or don't want to eat. You are mentally triggered by these negative thoughts to eat – especially accessible snacks. If these mental mind drainers do not make you eat more they may affect your desire to exercise. If your life is filled with any of the following emotions you are not likely to feel like exercising. You may be more prone to lie around and build up stress and anxiety that over a period of time will be very detrimental.

Fear

We live in an age of so much fear. People fear everything today. There is the fear of tomorrow. People fear what tomorrow will bring. There is the fear of death. What happens if the doctor diagnoses cancer? What will happen if my retirement income is not sufficient? What happens if my spouse leaves me?

There are truly some things we should fear like drunken drivers, rattlesnakes and muggers among others. But some people spend their lives being afraid of any and everything.

1 John 4:18 says this, "Fear has torment." When fear takes over a life there is no rest. You cannot concentrate on what is important. Your mind and life are preoccupied with what is scaring you. This becomes a form of torment. You need to exercise but it's hard to think about a work out because you are so mentally exhausted from fear. On the other hand, if you will exercise, some of the negative

energy that is storing up in your body will be released. A good aerobic walk or thirty minutes of some kind of good sweaty exercise will serve as a break to all the junk thinking that is clouding up your body and mind.

There are the quick fears of life. We see a car about to cross over into our lane on a busy highway. Rightly so, that scares us. The missed incident sends a shock wave through you and it may take you a mile or so down the road before your heart returns to normal.

The ongoing fear of life is what does us in. When we day after day have something that is about to tear our hearts out because there is an element of unknown as to what will happen. Maybe you lost your job and nothing seems to be opening up for you. There are bills that are mounting up and you may have children and a spouse that are dependent on you. That can be scary. Fear of your circumstances is tormenting you.

You may have made a mistake and the fear of your mistake is regretful and torments you.

Fear brings bondage. The Bible talks about a person in Romans 8:15 who all their lifetime is in bondage because of fear. I believe life is too short to live it in fear. Matthew chapter 25 in the Bible has Jesus relating a story about a man that was given a certain amount of money but out of fear he would not invest it…instead, he buried it because he was afraid.

Fear holds us back. You may not be the achiever in some realm that you ought to be because you have been shackled by fear. You are afraid you will make a mistake.

The Bible says in 2nd Timothy 1:7, "God has not given us the spirit of fear – but of love, power and a sound mind."

A sound mind is a healthy mind. A healthy mind is a functioning mind. A functioning mind controls the body.

You feel much more like getting out of bed and seizing the day when your mind is in right order. A fearful mind is a cloudy mind unable to fully give its best attention to what is best for one's life and body.

How do you deal with fear? You must face it with faith. Psalm 23, "Even though I walk through the valley of the shadow of death, I will fear no evil. You are with me. Your rod and your staff comfort me."

"When I am afraid I will trust in you," (Psalm 56:3).

"Perfect love casts out fear," 1st John 4.18. God loves us perfectly. It is not my perfect love but God's perfect love for me.

Resentment

Resentment is an ugly state of mind. Resentment toward anybody will hurt you. Normally, you are the only one that is hurt. The person you are resentful toward is often clueless about how you really feel about him or her.

Don't resent people who have more than you. It will not help you to have any more. Don't resent people whom you feel are more attractive physically than you. It does not make you any more attractive. Do not resent people who are more talented. It does not make you any more talented. Do not resent other's accomplishments. It does not accomplish anything for you.

Resentment only devours your energy. When you are using your emotions resenting someone then you are only depleting what you might have used to achieve a similar success.
Resentment depletes your resources of energy and mental clarity to accomplish life's goals.

Learn to admire people. Develop a sense of appreciating what others have been able to accomplish. It may be true that they seemingly have had more breaks or more help than what you feel you've had. But so often in life we make many of our opportunities.

There are cases of course when life seems impossible. Karen was a total invalid and could have taken the attitude that her life was totally useless. Yet, she found ways to encourage and bless the lives of her friends who visited with her. One friend would write down a couple of paragraphs of words from Karen that would appear in the church weekly paper. The first column that people read was the words from my wife. People were interested in hearing what she had to say. Her illness rendered her body to a state of where she could do nothing, yet she still managed to do so much. I can only imagine how easy it would be for me to be filled with bitterness and anger if I could no longer run, swim and do all the things I enjoy doing. I cannot imagine how I could handle it. I might be prone to be resentful of others who are able to do what I could not do. Yet, I know that life is dulled when we are envious or resentful. Our lives miss out on greatness when we degrade ourselves into little begrudging people. Karen was greater than I because she could deal with her invalid state and bless other's lives.

Again, admire and give thanks for the beauty of others. We should let their beauty spur us to be more beautiful. We should let the physical fitness of others challenge us to take better care of our bodies. What others have accomplished should remind us that all things are possible. Christopher Reeve will never play Superman on television again, but he will always be Superman in the way that he encouraged so many people through his outward attitude. Nancy Reagan will never again reside in the White House of the United States as the First Lady of our country. Yet, she led our nation in her role model as a caregiver to President Ronald Reagan as he suffered with Alzheimer's. People whose lives are distraughtly changed can be overcome with resentment that zaps the very flow of life's energy from them.

Resentment will do to you what sand does to machinery. It grinds away at you. You are no longer able to perform and live calmly and smoothly.

Proverbs 15:17 "Better is a dinner of herbs where love is than a stalled ox and hatred therewith." In other words a peanut butter sandwich is much better than the best and biggest steak if you and your wife are arguing at the dinner table. No matter how sumptuous the meal you've not enjoyed it.

Jesus said in Matthew 5:44, "Love your enemies. Bless those who curse you." You ought to do this because it's right. Next you should do this because it pays. A friend of mine who is a psychologist has said that if you love God and love your neighbor you are not likely to have mental illness.

One man was talking to his minister and he said, "There are some folks I can't love," and his pastor said, "Sir, there are some folks I can't love, but there is no one Jesus cannot love. And Jesus is in us. The love of God is shed abroad by the Holy Spirit. Sometimes we have to step back and let the Lord love that person through you. You don't have to love what they do. But a general overall day in and day out attitude of resentment toward anybody will begin to wear on you and hurt you.

Don't go to bed with resentment or anger. You go to sleep every night with resentment and or anger toward someone and it depletes your energy. You don't sleep well. In the morning time you don't feel like taking your three-mile walk or run because you have wrestled all night with resentment. There is no peace and it physically catches up with you.

Inferiority

The feeling of being less than others is a horrible feeling and can cause emotional problems. This is why some people have such a need to belong to organizations.

People get themselves into financial problems because they need esteem.

One woman who could not balance her checkbook and was in financial trouble said, "It's the neighbors' fault. They keep buying things I can't afford."

Why does a person take drugs? He drinks a lot of liquor, smokes a few joints and he feels ten feet tall.

But we don't need to create financial problems for ourselves, or use harmful drugs. We are all special people that God has made. We are all different. But difference does not mean that anyone is inferior to another. You can take whatever God has given you and maximize it to the very fullest. If you are five feet tall quit fretting that you are not 5'10. If you are 7'0 you cannot be 6'0. There are some things in life that you cannot change. If you were born to parents that did not have large incomes and were not able to give you everything that you would have liked, move on. Make the best of whatever you have and build on it.

We compare ourselves to other people. We say he has better genes or she has longer legs or he has stronger shoulders or she has more beautiful hair. When we compare ourselves we get this inferiority complex. This is when we draw back. We are afraid to go to the gym and exercise because we feel from the outset that we are sub par and we shrink back. We rob ourselves of doing something positive because we allow the negative in us to control us.

"I can do all things through Christ who strengthens me," Philippians 4:13. You are who you are and you are wonderful. God has not made you to shrink back into a hole because you feel less than others. God wants you to take hold of this day and do something great for you! That may be paddling a canoe with your best friend or children or riding a bicycle around your subdivision. Christ will give you strength to seize the opportunity of living!

Guilt

David said in Psalm 51 that he was literally sick over his sins. He felt so bad that it felt like his bones were aching. He would go on to confess his sins and not blame them on somebody else. He would also pray for cleansing and he would consecrate himself to God to do better in his life.

In 1st John chapter one we read, "The blood of Jesus Christ God's Son cleanses us from sin."

Two wounds that are very harmful to the human psyche are sorrow and guilt. Sorrow is a wound that time will heal. Guilt is a dirty wound that festers. Guilt stems from transgressions, but you don't have to become sick over guilt. David dealt with his problem by confession, praying for help, cleansing and recommitting and changing his life to do better.

Guilt can rob a person of a happy life. Even David prayed and asked God to restore his joy. He had lost all joy about his life. But when you make a mental commitment to deal properly with whatever is dragging you down then you are on the road to wellness and life fitness.

Either of the four of these emotions and feelings can drag us down in our daily lives. They are internal matters of the mind and soul that must be properly cared for. Grinding fear, resentment, inferior feelings and agonizing guilt are matters of the inward life that will affect how you treat yourself. Life fitness for mind and body are worthy goals but these mental conditions afflict our success.

Suggestions:

1.   Take your life before God daily in prayer. He loves you and wants to help you. Talk to Him about what you are dealing with.

2. Exercise in some form at least five to six days a week. Your workout for the day may be mowing the grass or working in your shrubs or flower garden. It may be cleaning your house. But do something that gives your body a chance to release whatever is going on inside. For me it means doing something that allows my body to break a good sweat. There is something about sweating that purifies the body.

3. Make one or two good friends. A person of too many friends will come to ruin. Why? Because it's impossible to maintain ten or fifteen really close friends. But two or three close friends are healthy. You may meet them at church, a school function, they could live down the road or they could be people that you find in exercise clubs. Every body needs somebody to talk to. People pay huge amounts of money to talk to psychologists when maybe all they need is a friend to listen for just a little while.

4. Worship every week. There is a hole within us that only God can fill. Gathering with other people every week to worship Him is a mental and spiritual lift that every life needs.

5. Make a daily effort to do your best at whatever you have to do.

6. Plan time for you every day. It's your life too! We live much of our lives caring for children, parents and jobs and other commitments. Make sure your schedule has figured in some time to take care of you. Who else is going to if you don't?

7. Do the right thing daily. Don't violate yourself. Violation of what you know to be good and right only allows for the negative emotions of fear, guilt and even inferiority.

Violation is a tearing down of yourself that only allows for feelings of resentment toward others who seem to be doing it right.

8. Love God and love your neighbor. As you care for yourself and love the creator who made you don't forget to be kind to others. A gesture of kindness a day from every human being can only make the world a better place to live.

Chapter 17

Is Life Fitness Easy?

Our attitude determines much of what is easy and hard. Driving a car may be hard when one begins to learn, but soon the driver sits down underneath the wheel and drives without fretting about it being difficult.

Learning the keyboard in a typing class may begin with frustration. But, within a couple of months the typist is moving his fingers with the greatest of ease.

Baking came easy for my mother. At least it seemed to me that it did. She knew exactly what to do and went through the motions with the greatest of ease to put a feast on the table. Cooking is much more of a job for me. I don't have much practice or much of a commitment to kitchen excellence however; I'm kind of like many people who think about exercising. I have intentions of doing better in that area.

Fitness is a mind game that usually is a mind over matter scenario. To say that it's easy to get up every morning and utilize the first section of your day for exercise can be a challenge. I say the first section of your day because I don't think a person should necessarily jump out of the bed and begin exercising. The first thirty minutes may be your best time to sit down for a nutritious snack, a note pad and your Bible and have a little quiet time. I think the body feels more like exercising if it has had a few minutes to wake up and become alert. Plus you have mentally allowed yourself to make note of some of the important tasks to be done for the day.

Everybody is different in some respects. It may be that you meditate better and feel more like charting out your daily activities after your workout. Do what is healthy for you mentally and physically. The main thing is that you do the things that are important. You don't have to get locked into the thinking that if you don't read your Bible the first jump out of bed that you are not spiritual or that you are doing something wrong. Mental fitness is about being unshackled and living in the freedom that God has given to us. Your best contemplation may come at the noon hour. Do what is best for you and only you know what is best.

How is Fitness Hard?

Life is hard when our way of living is radically changed. When I was child we did not have air conditioning. I do remember sitting in front of the fan as a kid. I also remember trying to shower and leave the house looking decent in 95-degree high humidity weather. That was a challenge! But at the time it didn't seem so bad. It was hot – such was life. We were glad for cooler temperatures but life didn't stop because of the heat. Today I am air conditioned – conditioned. I am conditioned to air conditioning. When it's 95 degrees outside I want the air conditioning on. If I am showering to clean up for the day I don't want to be sweating by the time I have my clothes on. I don't mind sweating during a workout but I don't want to prepare for a meeting or to go out with people in a humidity-filled 95-degree house. I'm used to air- conditioning because of the many years that I have now enjoyed it. A change back to a non air-conditioned house would be tough.

Life is hard when we make dramatic changes. A move to another city is stressful. Changing jobs is never easy. Divorce can be excruciating. Remarriage can present some incredible challenges. Going away to college or dropping your child off at college knowing that life will never be the same is a tough challenge. When I saw my oldest son Jared walking into the Navy recruiter's office to go off to boot camp I sobbed and cried most of the afternoon. Change is always hard...but the only constant in life is change. Life will change for you whether you do anything or not.

Your body is aging and it needs attention. A car can be driven a long time but it needs constant care. Sometimes it needs major repairs such as new transmissions and motors. Those kinds of major overhauls are painfully expensive. Our bodies require services throughout life. However, hopefully routine maintenance may prolong the life and health of your body just as routine maintenance does your car. A major repair to a car is hard and so are major body repairs.

Being inattentive to your body can become a very slothful way of living. Anyone can become accustomed to ignoring the needs of his or her body. Life can be lived without any exercise, lack of rest and poor eating choices. It can be a way of life and sadly is for many Americans. The thought of changing is hard. But right thoughts lead to right choices. Getting your mind to where it should be is the first step.

Beginning the commitment to actually eat differently and exercise is hard because it means change. But the key to change is allowing it the time to become routine to you. Don't quit the third day when your body is screaming for a candy bar. Eat the candy bar...but then resume your forward commitment to fitness. You can't eat candy two or three times a week and have success in your fitness program. You may be fortunate if you can have a candy bar once a week. Saturday may be your day that you go for a small dessert, maybe a scoop of vanilla ice cream, if you have had a good week eating and exercising. Condition yourself to this kind of change and it will become a way of life. It's mental. Fitness is a mind game.

How is Fitness Easy?

Life is easier when our attitude is that life is different. Difficulty is based more on perception than on reality. We make life hard when we refuse to adjust. An unwillingness to be bendable or flexible will only cause you to break. The person that cannot roll with the punches of life will more quickly shatter into pieces. It's not a perfect world and life changes. People change and circumstances are always changing. It bugs us to no end sometimes but it's life. And the quicker we can adjust the more rapidly we can move on with a healthier frame of thinking.

Fitness begins to shape our lives when we determine to make adjustments and allow them to make our lives better. We go for the change that is good for us and reap the rewards of sticking with the positive change.

Fitness becomes a lifestyle. It's easy because that's how we have chosen to live. Once the choice has been made then every day we know how we are going to live, eat and conduct our bodies and lives for the maximum benefits. We know that we are going to get in our exercise and that we are going to be careful about what and how we eat. It's not a miserable feeling. We eat but we do it with control. A car going down the interstate at 65 mph is fun. But if it is out of control it becomes a ride of terror. The airplane under control is enjoyable but when it becomes out of control then the plane ride is one of horror.

Life is to be lived under control. Fitness is taking control of your life and making the ride as smooth as you can make it. You have to make changes that at first seem to make your life miserable but you adjust, and your life and body begin to show the rewards of your new attitude toward life. If you go in the ditch then get out of the ditch. Evaluate why you went into the ditch and then proceed forward and try to avoid the ditches. If you hit an air pocket as in a plane ride then settle down and proceed forward. There are always bumps, ditches and air pockets along the way. Being derailed momentarily doesn't have to be forever. Count your loss and keep going. Staying in the ditches of life is when life becomes hard. Take the attitude that you will drive your life with more control and try to avoid the next ditch around the corner. And when that ditch comes along you pass right by it and keep going because you have already decided to avoid going into it before you ever come close to it. You have made the mental decision to make your ride smooth, easy and controlled. Life fitness is easy because it is a choice that you make.

Chapter 18

Think A Happy Thought

Our thought lives control our actions and without the right thinking we are not going to produce the right behavior.

The movie Hook starring Robin Williams is a movie based on the fairy tale Peter Pan. In the movie Peter Pan loses the ability to fly. His flying ability has been thwarted by his downcast feelings. His ability to fly comes back to him when he is able to think a happy thought. When he thinks happy thoughts he is able to soar through the air. While it's only a movie and a fairy tale there is some very innate truth to the story line. We fly or we crawl as we think within us.

Think a happy thought. Think good thoughts. Think positive thoughts. Think hopeful thoughts. Think possibility thoughts. Be a believer.

If you look for the negative you will find it. If you look for an excuse you will find one. If you want to think ugly thoughts you can think them all day. Ugly thoughts make for an ugly person and unhappy thinking makes for unhappy living. Plus, they keep you from flying. They keep you walking – barely. Truthfully, your walking becomes more of a limp, a slow dragging kind of crawl.

How many people go every day with the attitude, "I'm just barely getting by.", or "I'm just barely making it."? The more they dwell on the word "barely" the more barely their life really is. The person who says life is bad and keeps saying life is bad only makes life worse. The person who says life is good and keeps believing that life is good will only make his life better. It's not the idea that you are trying to fool yourself. But happy thoughts lead to more positive actions. There is more energy to move, produce and have quality action about your life. Because you believe! You believe in you. You believe in God. You believe in what is the very best!

1 Corinthians chapter 13 in the New Testament is credited as being the love chapter in the Bible and truly it is! This chapter tells us about all the good qualities that are the result of positive inward thinking. Love is a very incredible upbeat positive emotion. Love is a happy thought. Hate is an unhappy thought. Love is an upward thought. Dislike is a downward thought.

In love we soar. In bitterness or anger we go to the miry pit of despondency where no one is flying or thriving. A loving family is a flying family. A fighting family is one that is limping and crawling along trying to survive and often does not.

Successful people are those who are able to love and be loved.

Families that arise above the trials of life are families that have love and work through their problems.

The person who is able to take hold of life and push to greater excellence knows love is essential. There must be love for self. You can't love others if you do not love yourself.

Love believes. Love hopes all things. Love sees the best in others. Love endures. The scripture says there is faith, hope and love but the greatest of these is love.

The concept of all three of these is upward and positive. It is thinking upward, heavenward and seeing the best in life and in others.

This kind of attitude gives you a lift like nothing else. It's a faith lift, hope lift and a love lift. When you are lifted by faith, hope and love then you have no choice but to soar. We aren't like the birds. The birds were truly made by God to fly. Yet, as human beings we can soar in how we approach our daily lives.

When you are filled with faith, hope and love you can hit the road doing your two or three- mile walk or run. You make it to the gym to do those important weight resistant exercises. You don't have to have the biggest meal on the menu and then the biggest dessert when you eat out. You are already happy. You don't have to feed your body with everything in the restaurant to be happy. Your happiness is not dependent on doing negative things to your body that will only make you feel worse. Your happiness is internal. Internal happiness enables you to fly over those negative hurdles that only trip us up and make us feel worse.

Keep Believing

Believe that it is possible. Whatever it is that you want to do, you are more likely to do it if you believe.

Hope is a wonderful quality of life. When we lose hope we give up. Wherever there is hope there is a willingness to keep trying.

Have faith. Without faith we feel hopeless. When we lose faith despair sets in and we go into neutral waiting for the worst to happen. Remember our ultimate faith is in God who has made us. His power and strength are like nothing else.

There are some things in life that we cannot change. It is a fact that we will all die. Some day by disease or disaster, but we will all die. There comes a point when the body cannot be turned around and saved and death comes. Death is not the end for the believer. Jesus promised eternal life to every believer. In heaven God has prepared a marvelous place for all of His children. Yet as long as there is life, there is hope until we totally give up. When we give up then real life is over.

Love is like nothing else. Love keeps us working, trying and doing the best we can possibly do. Love does for the heart what nothing else can do. This emotion gives us a lift and enables us to fly.

Think a happy thought and it will lift you. Keep thinking them and you will fly. Fill your life with belief, faith and love and you will soar in heavenly places.

Isaiah the prophet has these incredible truths, "He gives strength to the weary and increases the power of the weak. Even youths grow tired and weary, and young men stumble and fall; but those who hope in the Lord will renew their strength. They will soar on wings like eagles; they will run and not grow weary, they will walk and not be faint," (Isaiah 40: 29 – 31). How can we ever possibly wait upon God with all the adversity and trials that we go through in life? Because we believe, we hope, we have faith and love. These enable us to soar, even when life is unsuitable for flying.

Chapter 19

Stop The Craziness!

You cannot lose weight if you eat all the time. You cannot experience life fitness if you always have food in your hand. Stop it!

Crazy Living

A sure sign that your life is out of control and that you are headed for obesity or trapped in obesity is when you cannot pass a fast food restaurant. Of course you pass many of them because you can't stop at them all. But two and three times a day you find yourself thinking only of one thing and that is-which fast food restaurant do I stop at next for some junk food? When junk food eating becomes a lifestyle you are living a lifestyle that can only mean excess weight and lots of it.

Convenience stores are readily available today. They are on every corner throughout much of America. A Convenience store provides a speedy outlet for candy bars, cakes, pies, sugar filled soft drinks, chips, fat filled hot dogs and on and on. A meal of a soft drink, a small bag of chips and a candy bar and you are doomed for the day. You are talking about 30 grams of fat in this tiny snack not counting all of the sugar from the soft drink. Plus, with all three items together you are looking at six hundred calories of very non-nutritious food. You might get by with this every two or three weeks but you can't do it daily. It's not a good idea even weekly. You are trying to get into shape – why do it to yourself? Life fitness is about balance. But there is nothing balancing about putting sheer trash into you body.

Dangerous living is when you just live every evening from

six until bedtime running back and forth to the refrigerator. Find something else to do other than eating all the time. Seriously, doesn't it seem crazy to constantly have something in your mouth for two and three hours all evening? And then you look in the mirror and you fuss about it. You fuss about how you look. You complain about your clothes and how they feel. You complain that you feel bad in summer clothes. Well, stop the craziness! Stop eating all the time!

Surely, eating is important and we should eat every day. We should eat three, four or five times a day. But they should be small portions of food that are healthy. You are not to eat three big meals a day. If you do you will be as big as the side of a country barn, unless you are blessed with an incredible body that burns it away. Bodies with these kinds of metabolisms are few and far between it seems. I'm not talking about starving yourself. You don't have to starve yourself. You may eat. And you may eat well. But you cannot eat all the time. If you get on a diet that tells you that you may eat all you want all the time then likely it's someone that has a lot of food to sell! They are not in the fitness business; they are in the food selling business! You cannot eat all you want all the time. You may eat someone's product for breakfast, lunch and dinner. If the products you are eating have between 300 and 500 calories each and you eat nothing else you are likely to reduce your weight. If this is what it takes for you then so be it. I'm for people doing whatever it takes to get their bodies and lives into shape as long as it is within reason and utilizes sane and healthy procedures.

Starving yourself to death is not the way to go either. However, I repeat - be careful of diet groups who have all kinds of food products they are pushing your way. The grocery store will have what your body needs to eat. You don't have to buy expensive foods from fitness groups in order to reduce your weight. If this does it for you mentally and gets you kicked into gear to lose weight then that is what you need to do. But learn to shop a little smarter at the grocery and you can provide your body with the same kinds of nutritious food, as you would buy from an expensive fitness organization.

Again, be careful of anyone who tells you that if you buy their food, you may eat all that you want. Be careful of diet planners who tell you that if you follow their plan, you may eat all that you want. This is exactly what we want to hear. We want to believe that we can go to the pig's trough, eat like pigs but not look like pigs! We want somebody to tell us this. We want to be convinced of it. We want to be able to just lie in our lazyboy chairs every night and feed our faces until we are blue in the face the entire time saying, "I'm on this new diet. It's a great diet. I can eat all I want on this diet." Of course you can. You can eat all you want all the time on any diet. But go and check your scales and see how much weight you have lost. See if you really have lost inches and if your dress or jeans feel any better or looser on you. Stop the craziness! The only way that you can eat a lot is if you are really exercising hard and working out a lot, even then you still have to be meticulous in your eating. If you are running five miles every day you may very well be burning close to a 1000 calories. However, what is 1000 calories? One thousand calories is one Big Mac and a small order of fries. That's it! You would be better off to run one mile and leave off the Big Mac and fries. You would save yourself a lot of time. Do you really have the time in your life to be so wasteful?

I see people all the time who run five miles so they can eat a junk food meal. I wonder if they don't have anything else to do. They could have saved themselves the hour of time if they had just been more careful about their eating. If you eat correctly you will get far more results from your exercise program. Exercising all the time and eating all the time gets you nowhere but frustration.

I can hear somebody saying now, "I just love to eat, so I

exercise all the time." If you have nothing else to do with your
life but to live on a treadmill, hang out at the gym and constantly
exercise three hours a day then go for it. But, chances are you may
want more for your life. You may have children. You may have a
spouse or other loved one. You may have a job or career that you
need to invest time in. Allow yourself time for life, love, family, and
career by not having to live a life of constant exercise! Again, I can
hear someone saying, "I love to exercise." Then, so be it. If that is
your passion and love then that is your passion and love. If you are a
fitness person whose career is the gym then you may very well have
sane reasons to dedicate your life to a gym or clocking multi hours of
running on the road. But the average person is someone who wants
to lose some weight, feel better, get into his or her clothes and have
a healthier life. The way to do this is to stop eating all the time and
exercise five or six days a week.

Out of Control

Our lives tend to swerve off the road. We are not able to live on
automatic pilot for very long. To this day I cannot turn loose of the
steering wheel of my car and take a nap. I cannot trust my car to stay
on the road. For some weird reason if I let go of the steering wheel
my car will run into the ditch, a curb or hit an oncoming vehicle.
It's dangerous to let go of the steering wheel! An out of control car is
a dangerous car.

An out of control life is a dangerous life. It's dangerous to you
and it's dangerous to the people who need you at home and at work.
When you are out of control eating everything you can get your
hands on and keeping something around for a snack all the time you
have lost sight of what your life is about. You are out of control. Your
life is headed for disaster. You will become so sluggish that you don't
feel like going to work. You will not feel like mowing your grass or

doing your dishes. You will have energy for nothing. All you will want to do is sit or lie on the couch or live in your bed. You then are hurting others. You have family or friends who need you and need the contribution that you can make to their lives. You are letting them down. You are failing them because you will not gain control of the steering wheel of your life and take charge of yourself.

You may do a good job at work. But truthfully, you know you could offer far more if you felt better. If you had more energy you could be more productive.

When life consists of mindless out of control eating you are headed for an early grave. Or, a life robbed of many opportunities. Do you want to be on oxygen when you are sixty years old because you would not gain control of your eating? Do you want to be taking disability from your work when you are fifty-five because you are too fat to work or be productive? What a poor excuse to take disability. "Mr. Employer my doctor tells me I am disabled because I'm as fat as a bear and therefore I can't get my breath and therefore I can no longer work and be productive." Basically what you are saying is that emotionally you are disabled. Anyone who takes their life to this point, where they are disabled because of their eating, is emotionally out of balance. They have totally turned loose of the steering wheel of their lives to the point of disaster. They have utterly ignored their bodies and health and what is the very best for their personal lives. They have been abusive and destructive to themselves.

Self abuse and self-destruction is a sad reality of life. We see it all the time. People smoke themselves to their death. People drink alcohol to their death. People do drugs to their death and people eat themselves to their death. Don't point your finger at people who smoke and drink alcohol if you refuse to stop eating like a hog and looking like one.

I know I'm coming down hard in this chapter and there may be someone who has a medical thyroid condition that has greatly contributed to the physical shape they are in. There are medicines that will cause you to put on mega pounds of weight. Talk to your doctor. Tell your doctor you want your medicine changed. Tell your doctor that it's not fair for you to have to battle weight that this insane medicine has added to the body that you care about.

If you have a medical condition that is keeping you fat, then talk to your doctor. If you need medical help then please go for it. If you don't, then all this excess weight you are carrying is only going to do more health damage to you. You have a life. There are people who need you. God wants your life to be productive. But you can't be productive if your life is out of control.

Chapter 20

Basic Plans for Daily Fitness
Life Fitness Planning Pad is Vital!
Or, Eat Six Meals a Day!

A single plan is not for every person. But without a plan you are bound for failure. Every life needs a daily plan of action. I repeat, a daily plan. You can't decide to be fitness minded one day a week or month. Life fitness is daily. Even on the days when you eat a little more, you have planned for it because, six days prior, you built it into your weekly fitness plan.

A fitness plan for every day and week is a plan for success. Buy a Life Fitness Planning Pad. The planning pad is that very important pad where you write down every week what you intend to accomplish the next week. You will refer to it weekly, daily and some days, maybe hourly. The planning pad has the list of objectives you are trying to achieve for the day and even for the week.

Plan for fitness. Plan for life. Plan for family. Plan for career. Plan for retirement. Nothing is set in concrete and plans are always apt to change. But without plans there is little to no chance for success.

A Plan for a Week

Plan out your Sunday through Saturday. Begin the Thursday or Friday before Sunday. Begin to make notes as to what kind of week you would like to have. Again, it's the week you would like to have. You are considering in this schedule what you would like to accomplish plus you are making decisions about what you will try to accomplish. Also, you are charting down your exercise pattern or routine for the week. You are making plans to have a successful week because when the week starts you will know what you expect to do for the next seven days. You have a plan! When Sunday comes there will be none of this, "I don't know what I'm going to do. You do, because you have made the plan.

Remember, you are working on your plans before Sunday begins for the weeklong planning effort.

Sunday – This is the first day of the week. What do you normally do on Sundays? You will need to decide which day this week you will allow yourself to eat with a more relaxed attitude. I strongly suggest Sunday or the end of the week like Saturday. One day for a relaxed eating day is all your body can stand especially if you are just starting out on a fitness routine. This could be the day that you eat a sumptuous lunch or dinner. You may go for steak, fish or chicken with the extra vegetables. You can even splurge with a bowl of vanilla ice cream. But beware of those big desserts that are large enough to feed three people. You are just setting yourself up for extra grief. You could spend an entire day or two just trying to rid your body of this sweet disaster!

If Sunday is your day to eat pancakes, eggs, bacon, biscuits and then a large dinner, you need to be sure that you know where you are headed on Monday. On Monday, you can't have all that you ate on Sunday. Nor can you eat like you did on Sunday the rest of the week. Why? Because you are headed for life fitness and you are losing weight and getting your life into shape! You are going to be awesome! You have a plan and a goal. You can do it and you can live it!

Make Sunday a day for worship. We live in an age where there is much Saturday night church. Adjust your calendar as is best for your family. However, set aside time for worship of God. Begin your week with at least one hour of worship. God made you. He knows all about your body. He is a source of strength for you for the rest of the week. Spend some time with Him. You will find this a valuable investment of your time.

Sunday may also be your day for no exercise. Whatever we do in life requires us to step away from it. Regardless of how much you love exercise, fitness and sports it will become old to you if you do not take a break from it.

So here we are on the first day. What are we doing? We are eating, worshiping God and taking a break from exercise. How do you like this plan so far?

Monday – Put on the shoes you bought for walking or exercise. Comfortable shoes are important. Take care of your feet and they will take you places.

Walk a mile if you can. Only you know how much you can take.

If you are walking a mile in your neighborhood mark it off with your car by driving around the block. The odometer will tell you exactly where a mile is in your community. Make it your goal to go for the mile. If you are carrying a couple of extra hundred pounds then walking a mile will likely be way too much for you. Go for the half-mile.

Exercise works better at different times for different people. The morning may or may not be your best time. If you work on Monday, you may either have to exercise in the early morning or after work. However, on your planning pad write down exercise for Monday. Write down what time you are going to exercise. Write down exactly what your goal for exercise is. Your goal will be walking the half-mile or mile. You may be a little farther ahead in physical shape. It could be that running the mile may be more your goal. On your planning pad you are writing down that your goal is the mile run for Monday.

Eating goal for Monday – Plan for six meals! You can walk a mile anywhere from twelve to twenty minutes. Everybody is different. The purpose of life fitness is not to judge you for how fast you run a mile. Everybody would like to run a mile in less than five minutes but those days soon pass. Or, they may never have been in existence!

Whatever exercise you do on Monday can be nullified by your eating. You will lose anywhere from 100 to 200 calories when you walk or run a mile. It all depends on your body and how hard you walk or run. The treadmill tells me I'm burning off 170 calories when I run a mile. Some books say 200 calories are burned when you run the mile. It all depends on how much you move your arms when you are walking/running and how fast you go. Harder work will likely mean a greater burn of calories, but generally, you can safely figure between 150 to 200 calories burned. So if your calorie burn for Monday is about 200 calories then figure how much you are allowed to eat for the day.

If a 1500 calorie a day eating plan enables you to lose weight then walking or running one mile will not allow you to eat 2000 calories. You might be able to eat 1600 calories on this day but this is the max if you are serious about weight reduction.

For breakfast try a bagel with your favorite jam. An eight-ounce glass of orange juice and some water is a good start for the day. The bagel, jam and juice will add up to about 300 calories.
Coffee is not the best beverage of choice. If you are a coffee addict try to immediately cut down on your coffee intake. Five cups of coffee a day is way too much. Aim for three cups a day at first with your goal of cutting your coffee intake to two cups in the morning. Eventually you can go to one. In time you may be totally free from your coffee addiction. Caffeine is not good for your body. Soft drinks and coffee packed with caffeine are not the dieter's drinks of choice. You can drink them – but very sparingly. Ultimately, you are the healthiest if you can become caffeine free.

Try a mid-morning snack. This may be a banana, grapes or an

apple. One hundred to two hundred calories are enough for this time of the day.

For lunch try a health food bar. There are many good nutritious health food bars on the market. Go to your local health food store and shop for bars that provide protein and some carbohydrates. I prefer the bars that have some carbohydrates because I am exceedingly active and need the energy. I do strongly recommend you look for a blend bar. A blend bar will have a good mixture of protein and carbohydrates. A bar that is very heavy on the carbohydrates and low on the protein is not what your body needs either. These bars may be close to a regular candy bar if they are filled with sugar and carbohydrates. This could end up turning to pure fat by the end of the day if you are not very active.

A blend bar may have as many as 200 to 300 calories. A glass of water or decaffeinated beverage at lunchtime is all you need. Big high carbohydrate lunches only make for a high boost of energy that will likely drop you by 2:00 and your body will be crying for a nap. Do you really want to go back to work or back to your afternoon routine dying for a nap? No...you want your day to have energy and big lunches only zap your energy level for the afternoon.

The mid-afternoon meal should be very similar to the mid-morning meal. Again you are trying to keep this meal to 200 calories or less. Three slices of thin sliced ham are only about 100 calories with ten grams of protein! A caffeine-free soft drink or some water and you have staved off your hunger urge!

The evening meal may find you a little hungry. This is the danger time for many. You've only eaten 900 or so calories. You ran a mile during the morning. You are hungry. You may even be starving. Plan this meal carefully. You can eat well. You may be able to eat 400 or 500 calories depending on what you ate during the day.

Try grilled chicken. The chicken alone will only be about 100 – 150 calories, depending on size and if you put anything on it.

Barbecue sauce and even a little honey mustard are not too high in calorie or fat content. Be careful and don't go too crazy on the sauce. You can even have two grilled chicken breasts if you want! Your vegetable can be steamed vegetables or green beans. There are different philosophies on eating baked potatoes. They are filled with carbohydrates and burn off slowly. Do not put sour cream or butter on it. Eat it plain. Add a small salad. A bowl of lettuce with a few other salad items added will be good for you and low in fat and calories unless you cover it up with dressing! Eat it without dressing! If you have to have dressing then use only fat-free dressing, but use it very sparingly. A spoon full or two at the most is all you need. If you cover your salad up with fat filled dressing you are only kidding yourself. You are loading it down with fat – that's what you are trying to lose. For extra fun eat a banana or have some grapes. Chances are you will have room for a small dip of vanilla ice cream an hour or so later for your evening snack if you wish. Your calorie intake will be at 1500 calories. Plus you ran or walked a mile for the first day! You have lost some weight! Don't bother weighing yourself the next morning…but if you do and followed Monday's plan you will be a little lighter on the scale!

Tuesday – You may feel a little hungry. Try two scrabbled eggs and two strips of bacon. Be sure you wrap your bacon in a napkin before you eat it. Wrapping it in a napkin gives it a chance to drain off the grease. For a special treat pour some honey on your bacon. If you want to be wild and crazy pour a little honey on your eggs and bacon! The eggs and bacon are providing protein and the honey a little charge of sugar and carbohydrates. You will feel like you have had something to eat! You may prefer a boiled egg. For mid-morning have a sliced carrot on hand. For lunch on this day you may want to go strictly with salad. I suggest a grilled chicken salad. You can buy these at most restaurants or grill the chicken yourself and cut in up into some lettuce. If you go light on the dressing you have only had 600 to 700 calories so far for your Tuesday. For mid-afternoon have an apple on hand. At the evening time you have 800 to 900 calories to enjoy between your dinner and later evening snack. You may have pasta if you want. But pasta is big in carbohydrates. If you eat a very large helping of pasta and add bread you can have 900 calories between the two very quickly. Have a very small portion of pasta and keep the bread to one breadstick or very small piece. Do not add butter.

On Tuesday – do your walk or run again. You could be sore from the day before! Stretching before and after exercise is a must to deal with sore muscles that have not been used in awhile.
Try going for the same distance you did on Monday. You are working for balance and consistency in your life. Consistency and balance will produce amazing results!
If you do your aerobic walk or run in the evening, then try a few floor exercises. Try a couple of push-ups. They may feel awful! They probably will if you haven't been doing any. Try to do five sit-ups. Remember you are establishing a pattern for your life. You are not in Army boot training camp. Nor, are you training for an athletic championship (well, not at this stage anyway), but what you are doing is establishing a pattern and a plan to your life.

Remember planning is essential. On Friday or Saturday before your week begins write out your plan. Plan for every day. Plan your exercise and plan out what you are going to try to eat throughout the day. If you don't do it for the week then plan out your next day before you go to bed at night. This way when you get up in the morning and you reach for your planning pad, the planning pad already has on it what you want to do for the day! You got out of bed with a plan!
Failing to plan is a plan to fail.

It's possible to arise early in the morning and chart out your plans for the day. But then you are spending part of your important morning time planning. This does not mean failure but you could be using this time having a quite moment with God, exercising or being creative. If you are an all day, fast paced person, it may be that you don't have anything left for exercise after six at night. By this time you have wound down. Yet, you are still able to think about what you did not do right during the day and how you might do life better the next day. This is where your planning pad comes into great use. You may be watching a little television or you are relaxing an hour or so before bedtime. You take out your pad and you make notes as to what you want to eat and what kind of exercise you want to do the next day. Of course you will want to include important dates, commitments, work and meetings that you may be obligated to on your calendar.

Wednesday – Do a different form of exercise. Do you have a bike? Get it out for a mile or two ride. If it's the right season push mow your yard – unless you have several acres to mow and then this is not a good idea. But you might push mow some of it. Or if you like to play golf try walking nine holes. Pull your cart. If these three don't work do some housework. Anything that is active and mobile is most important.

Any of the above activities may burn off three or four hundred calories. But who knows for sure. It all depends on how hard you work at them. Since there is such an unknown and you are trying to reduce your weight don't go above 1600 calories for this day. Chances are you easily worked off a 100 calories if you did some form of mobile activity. On Wednesday morning go for dry toast and some fat free spread or low in sugar jam. You'll consume 200 to 250 calories in two slices of toast and jam depending on how much you spread on your bread. At mid-morning try a health food drink. There are several good drinks on the market that provide you with a lot of protein and essential vitamins. At lunchtime try either a health food bar for 250 to 300 calories and for mid-afternoon try three slices of no-fat cheese. Three slices will have less than a 100 calories. At dinner/supper time keep it to some sort of lean meat. Baked or grilled fish would be an excellent choice. You can always add a little salad, green beans and corn and you've had a nice dinner.

At the end of the day reward yourself with some fruit, light salad, protein drink or bar. Always gauge your snacks for about 200 calories or less. Remember at this point of the day you have already had five small meals!

Thursday – make this day a little harder. Determine you are going to walk faster and a little farther. You may determine instead of running one mile that this is the day you move up to one mile and a half. You may run on an empty stomach since more fat is burned on an empty stomach than when you try running on breakfast. Personally, I have to have a small snack sometime before I run. At least an hour before I run I feel that I need half a bagel with some flavored spread or some toast to get me going for the day. Too many healthy senior adults talk about the value of eating breakfast every morning. This seems to be good advice.

For Thursday mid-morning have a boiled egg on hand. It will be a great 10:00 morning meal!

For lunch you may want to treat yourself by going out. You can go out and still do well on your fitness weight reduction plan. Grilled chicken salads can be found at most restaurants. Or, you can order a vegetable plate. Leave off biscuits. Have toast without butter if you must have bread. Stay away from the buffet, you will destroy what you are trying to accomplish. A fruit plate or any kind or baked or grilled items will be okay if you do not overdo the meal with other items such a potatoes and huge portions of other side items. Just because you exercised a little harder does not mean you want to self-destruct at lunch. You can keep it to 500 to 600 calories and still have a fun lunch! Since you had such a big lunch you may want to

skip the afternoon meal and just have decaffeinated coffee or bottled
water would be nice. For Thursday dinner go for a baked sweet
potato and just a pinch of brown sugar and very little if any butter.
One large sweet potato and you will have had enough for the day. If
you are hungry at eight o'clock at night then dry wheat toast is not a
bad choice.

Friday – Go for some whole grain cereal and fruit for breakfast.
For your mid-morning meal try a fat-free yogurt. At lunch if you
are dying for some red meat you might splurge by fixing yourself a
hamburger. If you eat out leave off the cheese and the mayo! Most
places put too much mayo on and it's loaded with fat. The cheese
is normally filled with fat too. However, look for someplace that is
not a greasy spoon. Some restaurants are worse than others when it
comes to serving your burger with so much grease! You can fix your
hamburger at home without frying it in grease. Bake it, or get rid of
the grease before you eat it. Try some lean roast beef or some other
kind of lean meat such as turkey, which are normally better choices
than red meat.

For the Friday afternoon meal you can be creative. Three slices
of cold-cut turkey rolled up will be a tasty spark to your afternoon!

Friday night is a good time to continue to exercise caution. You
can go out and have fun but be careful. Be watchful always because
weight can be added quicker than it can be taken off. Keep your
dinner reasonable! If your Friday night meal lasted later then leave
off this late Friday night snack.

For Friday exercise you need to do your one-mile or even two-
mile walk or run. You are on a mission. Don't lose sight of what you
are going to look like! In just a few weeks you are going to notice
such an incredible difference in how you feel and look that you will
never want to go back to what you left! You are going to have energy
and a better even more positive attitude than what you may have
ever had!

On Friday do some floor exercises. You are likely to be sore from the sets done earlier in the week. But, today is a good time to try again. Go for another five or six push-ups and do some sit-ups. This time try ten sit-ups or as many as possible.

Saturday – is a big day because you have to exercise, watch what you eat and plan all over again for the next seven days. On this day you will take your Life Fitness Planning Pad and your calendar and prayerfully think about your next week. On this day, you consider everything that you know you will do for the next seven days. You will interweave all that you have to do with planned periods of time for meditation/devotional time, exercise and balanced healthy eating!

When the week comes and goes you are going to be overwhelmed at how much you accomplished and how much weight you lost and how much better you feel about yourself and life! Your attitude is going to be more positive and your weekly life's accomplishments are going to be more than what you imagined possible!

Dining Out Tips

Ask for salad dressing on the side and dip your fork into your dressing and then into your salad. Do not worry about cleaning your plate. Eat only until your hunger is satisfied. Leftovers make great next day meals. Remember you are also paying for the atmosphere and convenience, not just the food.

Approach buffets and salad bars with caution. Survey the whole buffet before selecting. Often an entrée is a wiser selection. The average person should keep their sodium intake to 1,100 – 3, 300 mg per day. The average caloric intake for a man or a woman is 2000 calories. If you want to lose weight it is recommended that

the female maintain 1200 – 1500 calories per day and the male stay around 1600 – 1800. If you want to lose weight, you should stay on the lower end of the recommended daily servings. Good sources of protein are lean meats, fish, poultry, eggs, beans, brown rice and barley. Fat calories in your diet should not exceed 30%.
Fat has 9 calories per gram.

Recommended intake of calcium is 800-1000 mg per day. Approximately 3 cups of low fat milk contains 800-1000 mg of calcium.

(Welborn Clinic and Welborn Health Plans Eating Out Guide – 421 Chestnut St. Evansville, Indiana 47713)

Food Guide Pyramid

The Food Guide Pyramid is an outline of what to eat each day. This has been debated more today than ever before. The Pyramid is not a rigid prescription but a general guide that lets you choose a healthful diet that's right for you. The Pyramid calls for eating a variety of foods to get the nutrients you need and at the same time the right amount of calories to maintain a healthy weight. Please keep in mind that servings do not represent three trips to the buffet table with a plate in each hand. Six servings of bread and pasta do not mean three slices of bread and three helpings of lasagna. Servings are very small in comparison to what we have become accustomed to eating in America. You can't add ten slices of bread to your daily intake and lose weight unless that is all you are eating and then you are depriving your body of protein and needed vegetables. Remember it's all about balance and small portions. A couple of slices of dry wheat bread a day is normally enough to meet the demands of the standard food group requirement. Two to four servings of fruit a day does not mean a quart of strawberries and half a watermelon in addition to whatever else you are eating. Two to three servings of meat, poultry and fish can be accomplished in a couple of grilled chicken breasts or small steak. By the way you don't need the combo meal where you get chicken and steak or fish and steak unless you have eaten very, very little during the day!

Many restaurants these days offer combo meals with two and even three meats not counting the baked potato and salad! It's too much! Remember too much is not good. You'll end up wearing some of your meal on your hips, stomach, thighs and nice full round face! It's about balance and portions. When making dining selections, keep in mind that foods from all the food groups are essential…you just don't need them all at once and very little of each when you do eat them. If you become mind and soul conscious about what you are putting in your body then you will soon discover that you need less food per day than what you think and there will be days when it's impossible to hit all the food groups. If you have a full life of activity it's difficult to plan your life to where you are getting the exact amount of fruit and vegetables that is healthy for you. The idea is common sense. Have a little meat, a little fruit, some dairy products and a little bread. Keep the portions small. The food groups and their servings for an average daily intake are listed below:

Food Group
Number of servings

Milk, Yogurt and cheese Group	2-3 servings
Meat, Poultry, fish, dry beans, Eggs & Nuts	2-3 servings
Vegetable Groups	3-5 servings
(Note: corn and potatoes fall in the bread group)	
Fruit Group	2-4 servings
Bread, Cereal Rice and Pasta	6-11 servings

(Welborn Clinic and Welborn Health Plans Eating Out Guide
– 421 Chestnut St. Evansville, Indiana 47713)

Drink Water!

Eight glasses a day keeps the fat away!

Water suppresses the appetite naturally and helps the body metabolize stored fat. Studies have shown that a decrease in water intake will cause fat deposits to increase, while an increase in water intake can actually reduce fat deposits.

What happens is the kidneys can't function properly without enough water. When they don't work to capacity, some of their load is dumped onto the liver. One of the liver's primary functions is to metabolize stored fat into usable energy for the body. But, if the liver has to do some of the kidney's work, it can't operate at full throttle. Therefore, it metabolizes less fat. Fat then remains stored in the body and weight loss stops.

Chapter 21

Life Management

Everything has limits. You have to know your limits and listen to your body. Any exercise program has its limits. Life fitness is not about pushing your body to the limits. This book is about exercise management. The key to life is management and balance.

Managing your life means being in control. You are the one in control of what you do each day. You are not living your life based on compulsion or addiction but on management principles. Fitness is a mind game – one of mind management. You are controlling the calls for your eating and exercise life. You are not exercising based on what anyone else is doing. You are exercising based on what is best for you. Just because the neighbor runs five miles every day does not mean that is what you are supposed to do. Running a mile every day may do for you what you need because you are controlling your eating. Eating right and some exercise complement each other for success.

It's easy to get into eating frenzies. I confess I can eat five or six pieces of pizza at a time. Is that good for me? No. It's me out of control. I can eat most of a fresh pecan pie. Is that good for me? No. It's me out of control. When I am out of control then I am hurting me.

I have days when I feel like running five or six miles. I don't need to do that unless I feel like it. If my body says it's okay – then it's okay. But whenever I get into a mismanaged life I may be eating 3000 calories one day rationalizing that I will exercise it off later in the evening or the next day.

Rationalization is the first step to obesity and misery.

We rationalize and say, "I can eat this dessert because I'm going to walk a mile in the morning." Wrong. You can't eat that dessert because walking a mile will not even begin to burn those fat grams and calories off that you ate in that dessert.

A friend of mine used to say, "I can eat anything I want." He would proceed to eat two slices of chocolate cake or whatever else he wanted. That afternoon he would run six miles and most every afternoon after work he was running five, six and seven miles. Truthfully, he could not eat anything he wanted without running six miles or more in the afternoon to burn it off. Let's say he was averaging ten minutes a mile. He probably ran faster but just to round it off. That equals at least one hour or more of running. How long did it take him to eat two pieces of chocolate cake? Probably about fifteen minutes if he was eating really slow. Does that make sense to you? Does it sound right to spend fifteen minutes eating as much as a 1000 calories not including fat gram content because you know you are going to spend one hour of constant running that might burn off 1200 calories? What if my friend had just said, "I'm going to split a piece of chocolate cake in half. I will eat one-half. The one half will satisfy my sweet tooth craving. Plus it will only be a minimum amount of calories in comparison to two whole pieces. The one half will possibly amount to about 250 calories. I can run two good miles, which will burn off as many as 400 calories. Then I will have my cake and eat it too! A little bit of weight will have been lost. Plus, think of all the extra time that is left. At least 40 minutes of time to either pursue lifting some weights for strength conditioning or going fishing, golfing or bowling with your children or a friend or anything that might be good for you and fun!

The person who is in a vicious cycle of eating wrong and over exercising is a miserable person on the worst kind of treadmill.

1st This person feels awful. The body is out of whack because of eating too much. But the body is also in a poor state because of the constant beating of too much exercise. This person is eating too much and then going out thinking, "I now have to exercise all this food off." Two hours may be given to running and aerobic type exercise. And then, what is left? There is little energy or mental alertness left to dedicate to anything else. You are spent!

2nd Nothing else is accomplished. What does this person have left to give to his education, job, family, hobbies or other pursuits? The answer is nothing. He has really very little if any to give. This individual has shot his/her day eating the wrong foods and then trying to burn it off or get rid of it. Wasteful life! If this is you stop it now! You don't have time to enjoy anything else about life because you are on this addiction cycle of eating like a pig and then having to go out and exercise like crazy. Your housework does not get done. You have no quality time with others. Your career is short changed. Your life has become mismanaged.

3rd It can happen overnight! Mismanagement happens to us all! The holiday season comes along and we say, "I'm going to enjoy the holiday. This is one day I am not going to worry about eating too much." Food lines the refrigerator for several days. We find ourselves letting go. We rationalize, it's the holiday and we will burn it off when Thanksgiving or Christmas is over. But the sad reality is that we never totally got rid of all that we gained last Christmas season. If we add another five or ten pounds this holiday season and add it to last year's weight that we are still carrying then where does that leave us? It leaves us with misery. It has us spending January and February trying to burn it off again.

Why not just enjoy life to the fullest and stay under management! Keep your life managed! Don't kick the manager out of your life for three or four weeks a year because then it could take you all year to recover from all the body weight that you gained. This is a waste of your good mental state and time.

Eat balanced and managed and exercise a little every day. Then you will have more time for life, fun, friends, family, career and other pursuits. If you eat and exercise poorly, then all you will feel like doing is eating and exercising. There is more to life than eating all the time and then having to exercise all the time to burn it off!

Determine you are going to be the captain of your ship. Say at this moment, I will not eat more than I need so that I don't have to spend all my mental energy fretting about what I need to lose and all my physical energy trying to lose it! I will be balanced! I will be the administrator of this life. No one else is going to do it! With God on my side I have the internal, mental strength to control my life and destiny. Remember, "I can do all things through Christ who strengthens me," (Philippians 4.13).

Chapter 22

Portions!

People have become accustomed to eating too much!
Everything is too much and too big. Fast food restaurants want you
to super-size everything. When you go through the drive thru you
are asked if you want your meal super-sized. If you say yes then for
a few cents more you can have almost twice the fries and an extra
large coke. The fries within themselves may have forty to fifty fat
grams depending on where you eat.

Many restaurants make sure you leave feeling full with bread.
More and more restaurants put all you can eat bread on the table.
The salads are big. Baked potatoes are huge with hearty portions
of sour cream and butter. Truthfully we can't blame restaurants.
Americans go out to eat at restaurants that have the best and the
most food. If the portions are small then we don't go back. This may
be why we are the fattest Americans of all time. Never has there
been such emphasis on fitness and proper eating. Never have there
been so many obese Americans.

Americans eat out today more than any other generation. And
when we eat out we want to make sure we are getting our money's
worth. Henceforth, we get our money's worth and we wear it at the
waistline, hips, thighs and chubby cheeks.

The key to life fitness is portion. Portion affects everything we
do. You can eat a balanced diet but you can't keep going back for
more and more. Your plate of food has to show that you have some
common sense. When our plates are heaping over with food falling
off the sides we only show our true colors – that there are some areas
of our lives that are not under control. If we were under complete

control we would make our food selections with some control.

You may be saying, "But what happens if I have worked hard all day…have not had anything to eat and I'm starving." This is often a real scenario. But the problem with this scenario is that it is not any healthier or wiser. You should never go all day without eating. You should be eating a little all day. You should be hydrating your body with water all day. When you come to the end of the day you will likely want to eat a little more at five, six or whenever you eat. You may easily consume seven, eight or even nine hundred calories! If you grazed a little all day like a cow grazes off and on throughout the day then you won't come to the dinner table starved!

If you go all day without food and have had very little water then when the evening meal comes you are famished. You rationalize that you can eat with total recklessness because you have fasted all day. You eat without thought of what you are consuming. When it is all over you may have consumed 2000 or more calories and you feel awful.

You need your energy and strength during the day. You need to be able to think clearly. When you starve yourself all day you are depriving your body of vital nutrients to make it as productive as possible. Eat a little off and on throughout the day. Eat 200 to 300 calories in the morning. Eat another 100 calories at mid-morning. Have 250 calories for lunch. In the afternoon go for another 100 calories. At dinnertime you are not starved. You are able to eat. But you don't have to eat everything in sight. You may eat as much as 600 to 700 calories. With all of this eating you should still have room for a mid-evening snack of 100 to even 200 calories. Let's add it up. Morning, mid-morning, lunch, mid-afternoon, dinner and evening snack. We are talking about six meals in a day! Your calorie intake is from 1350 to 1550! If you are exercising twenty to thirty minutes a day and keeping your eating at this level then you are trimming down, looking good and feeling better!

Chapter 23

Pace Yourself

Buy a writing pad and call it your "Life Fitness Planning Pad." On your pad you will make notes that will seriously affect your life. The purpose of the Life Fitness Planning Pad is for you to weekly and daily pace your life. As the manager of your life you have to keep records. You pace your spiritual life, mental life and physical life. They are all tied together. Often, either of them can become disjointed and affect the rest of your life.

Pace and keep track of what you must do every day. The planning pad makes that possible. You chart out your to do list for your life. You worked on it before the week began but daily you look to your planning pad to see what your objectives are for the day. On your planning pad you have written your exercise objectives. These may change daily. You may add or subtract as is best for your body. Your eating goal is listed on your planning pad. You know what you are going to try to eat and each morning you work on what you want to eat less or more of for that day! Your spiritual life is not last. Before you begin calculating what your numbers are going to be for the day you have already read your thought or scripture for the day and you are asking each and every morning for God's help to have a wonderful, healthy, spirit-filled, productive and successful day.

You won't lose 25 pounds in a week or even two or three. But you can lose a lot in a couple of months. If you pace yourself, eat right, keep track of your eating and exercise proportionately five days a week you can lose up to 25 pounds in three months. Maybe more! It does not require you to starve yourself or exercise yourself into the grave. It requires that you do some weekly planning on your

Life Fitness Planning Pad and have daily and weekly goals. And, most of all pace your self! In a couple of weeks you are going to be excited and in three months you are going to be thrilled.

Chapter 24

Make Every Day A Great Day!

Make every day of your life a great day-because it is! You are reading this book.

The fact that you can read is a marvelous gift. If you are able to hold this book or any book in your hands and read you are blessed. There are millions of Americans who are not physically able to hold up a book. You are alive enough to read this! Therefore rejoice for the opportunity you are blessed with to listen to the radio, read and watch television.

If you were able to move your feet to the floor from bed this morning and put on your own clothes you should rejoice because millions of people cannot.

Whatever you are able to do give God thanks and utilize whatever abilities you have to the fullest.

Build on your abilities. Don't fret about all that you cannot do. Rejoice for all that you can do. Pursue what you are able to do and your life will be full. You don't have to have ten different talents to be useful. Nor do you have to have three different jobs to stay busy. One talent enables you to be very useful. One job of any kind can keep you very busy.

Every night give thanks for all that you have been able to enjoy and do during the day. Determine that the next day is going to be a great day. You are going to do whatever is humanly possible to make your day good. You will look to God and thank Him for the sunshine or the rain, the peace or the pain, the ups or the downs, the smiles or the frowns and a win or a loss.

It may all sound whimsical and wish-like but we normally determine if our days are good or bad. Bad things still happen to us.

Accidents happen or we receive negative mail or a phone call comes that we do not particularly want to receive. Very simply, we can't keep the rain or even the storms from coming. But when they do come we brace ourselves for the storm and with our eyes on God we hold onto Him. He is our rock and stability when storms of life come our way. He enables us to stand firm when it seems the unexpected trials might literally blow us away.

It is this stability that we have in the Lord Jesus that keeps us pursuing life and coming out on top regardless of how hard we fall or are shoved to the ground by whatever storm or negative force that may come our way.

2nd Corinthians in the Bible has this passage, "We are hard pressed on every side, but not crushed; perplexed, but not in despair; persecuted, but not abandoned; struck down, but not destroyed," (4:8).

A decision to make every day a great day comes in part from our mental plan to allow life to be as good as it can be. Life fitness is a mind game. A fit life is a life that works to achieve wholeness in body and mind. It is what we extend our minds and bodies to do daily. Life fitness is about weekly and daily sitting down with our planning pad and saying this is the direction of life that I am taking and this is how with God's help I will stay on course and achieve my destination.

Making every day a great day comes by having a weekly and daily vision for your life. You have a goal for your spirit and your walk with God. Your goal may be memorizing one verse of scripture a week. Or your goal may be to simply read one chapter from the Bible a day. Or your goal may be to attend worship faithfully. Write down these goals on your weekly planning pad.

Every day is a great day because you are in control of what and how much you eat. You are planning and determining daily what you are going to put into your body. You will not eat out of habit or compulsion. You will use food to enrich, bless and help your life to be strong and useful. You will not use food as a way to fill some void in your life or as something to do when you are feeling depressed or anxious. Food is a wonderful gift from God to nourish and strengthen our bodies.

Every day is a great day because with whatever physical abilities you have you are going to find ways to exercise and strengthen the body that God has given to you. If you do not use your body properly, care for and maintain it with diligence your body will decline to a state of ineffectiveness and inability. If you are disabled or handicapped by disease, birth or some accident use whatever part of your body that is still functional. If a part of your body can still do something then allow it to function and give God praise for what you can do! Plan weekly and daily to exercise your body. God gave it to you. Don't waste it.

Finally, do your best. No one has ever failed who did his or her best. There are no losers in the classroom of life whenever each student did his or her best. No player in the sports complex ever walks away a loser if he or she knows they did their best. Doing our best is simply being faithful. It is having commitment and objectives that are honorable to God. Weekly and daily we plan our lives out to do the very best we can. We will have many failures and steer off our intended path to success. But because we have determined where we are going we are able to steer our lives back onto our desired path.

If you haven't already, then make this very moment the beginning of your new life!

Say these words:

I have only this moment. Yesterday is gone. There is no promise of tomorrow. The best I can be I will allow to begin now. What I begin to do now will bring change tomorrow. The change that I see tomorrow will have happened because I allowed it to begin today!

www.ingramcontent.com/pod-product-compliance
Lightning Source LLC
Chambersburg PA
CBHW031208270326
41931CB00006B/472